BEYOND CHOLESTEROL

*Vitamin B$_6$, Arteriosclerosis, and
Your Heart*

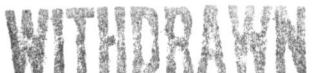

BEYOND CHOLESTEROL

Vitamin B₆, Arteriosclerosis, and Your Heart

EDWARD R. GRUBERG and
STEPHEN A. RAYMOND

ST. MARTIN'S PRESS • *New York*

For information, write: St. Martin's Press,
175 Fifth Avenue, New York, N.Y. 10010
Manufactured in the United States of America

Library of Congress Cataloging in Publication Data

Gruberg, Edward R.
　Beyond cholesterol.

　　1. Arteriosclerosis—Etiology. 2. Cholesterol—
Physiological effect. 3. Vitamin B_6—Physiological
effect. 4. Heart—Diseases. I. Raymond, Stephen A.,
joint author. II. Title. [DNLM: 1. Heart diseases—
Etiology—Popular works. 2. Arteriosclerosis—Etiology—
Popular works. 3. Homocysteine—Popular works.
4. Pyridoxine—Popular works. WG 113 G885b]
RC692.G78　　616.1'36071　　80-27745
ISBN 0-312-07779-3

Design by Dennis J. Grastorf

10 9 8 7 6 5 4 3 2 1

First Edition

Acknowledgments

WE ARE GRATEFUL for the help and encouragement of many people.

Moses Suzman came by our lab years ago and we first heard about the homocysteine theory from him. His enthusiasm ensnared, his story surprised. He led us to examine the assumptions of the cholesterol hypothesis and this eventually catalyzed us into writing our book.

One of the bonuses of working on this book has been getting to know Kilmer McCully. He generously gave us advice and suggestions at many stages of our manuscript. Our delightful conversations over lunch will long be remembered.

Betsy Altman, Eric Newman, Ann Northrup, and Bruce Reitz read and criticized many aspects of the manuscript. Sandra Raymond gave valuable support and criticism.

Fred Hapgood gave us practical advice about the vagaries of publishing and introduced us to Dick Todd of the *Atlantic* who recognized the importance of the homocysteine story.

Michael Binder enabled us to get a hands-on feel for arteriosclerosis.

Gerald Gaull told us about the early days after the discovery of homocystinuria and gave us some information that couldn't be culled from the published record. He also critically read our manuscript.

Tom Dunne and his staff at St. Martin's expedited the metamorphosis of the manuscript into a book. They made many useful suggestions for improving the text while not doing violence to the arguments.

We mined the resources of the Francis A. Countway Library

of Medicine. It is reassuringly complete, sensibly designed, and a fine place to work. The sub-basement room (which contains the Library's collection of journals published more than five years ago) has a characteristic mustiness that we won't forget.

Finally, we thank the many people who communicated with us over the last years with suggestions, information, queries, references, and criticisms (friendly and not so friendly). They sharpened our ideas and shaped our book.

Table of Contents

The idea of cause and effect is deriv'd from experience, which presenting us with certain objects constantly conjoin'd with each other, produce such a habit of surveying them in that relation, that we cannot without a sensible violence survey them in any other.

DAVID HUME

Introduction

OF ALL THE WAYS TO DIE, *arteriosclerosis* remains disquietingly popular. Fully one-half of the deaths in the United States this coming year will be the result of heart attacks and strokes, ailments that have their origin in the degeneration of blood vessels. Arteriosclerosis is a disease that impedes the vital flow of blood by causing arterial walls to thicken, harden, and eventually clog.

The medical advances of the recent past have provided effective cures for widespread communicable diseases, such as typhoid, cholera, and plague, and have completely eradicated smallpox. Together with nutritional improvements, the advances have made possible unprecedented population growth and a near doubling of the average human life span. Although work continues on the degenerative diseases, there is still no proven explanation for arteriosclerosis, and it remains the number one killer.

The reality of all the deaths creates an enormous need for some sort of explanation. Innumerable notions on the subject abound, though theories tying together many of the experimental and clinical findings are few. Worldwide research has produced so much data that it is quite intimidating to search the mountain of material for a coherent notion to suggest either cause or cure.

Today almost all Americans share with their doctors the same view of the disease that has held sway for more than 20 years. Arteriosclerosis is seen as arising from a variety of independent factors—cholesterol, stress, smoking, age, and sloth, among others. Evidence correlating each of these risk factors with the risk of coronary heart disease is plentiful. But the clinical and experimental record does not support the value of the established view as a guide to therapy. Low-cholesterol diets, for instance, consistently fail to lower blood cholesterol very much and they do not significantly reduce the risk of heart attack.

Most people who have arteriosclerosis do not look or feel sick. In a typical routine physical examination, an apparently healthy person will be told numbers for blood pressure (150/90, say) and *serum cholesterol* ("just above 200"). The patient knows that if these numbers are too high he probably has severe arterial disease. But high numbers are not perfect diagnostic indicators, and even people who forego butter, eggs, and chocolate mousse, who do not smoke, who exercise, and who have avoided stressful jobs can develop arteriosclerosis.

For those who have cardiac symptoms such as *angina* (chest pains), physicians prescribe tests to assess the narrowing of the coronary arteries. If the tests are positive, these people may undergo bypass surgery. Each year 50,000 people undergo such surgery. Surgery, though seeming to benefit individual cases, does not deal with the underlying arteriosclerosis. And recently some physicians are questioning the worth of coronary bypass surgery. What is clear is that everyone is susceptible to arteriosclerosis; pathologists report that nearly all Americans, even young ones, have some degree of the disease.

Not surprisingly, the state of medicine in regard to arteriosclerosis has prompted lamentations from physicians. The following appeared in the *New England Journal of Medicine*:

A generation of research on the diet-heart question has ended in disarray. The official line since 1950 for management of the epidemic of coronary heart disease has been a dietary treatment. Foundations, scientists, and the media, both lay and scientific, have promoted low fat, low cholesterol polyunsaturated diets, and the epidemic continues unabated, cholesteremia [blood cholesterol level] in the population is unchanged, and clinicians are unconvinced of efficacy. . . . This litany of failures must lead the clinician to wonder where the proper research and solutions lie. The problem of coronary heart disease is real enough here, and yet is rare in less developed societies. What aspect of life-style here makes atherosclerosis [a common form of arteriosclerosis] so malignant, its clinical consequences so fear-some?

George V. Mann, Sc.D., M.D. (1977)
Vanderbilt University

In the following pages we present a point of view at odds with the prevailing "risk factor" approach to arteriosclerosis. We believe that behind the risk factors lies an organizing principle, a single underlying mechanism that is affected by smoking, cholesterol, the passing of years, and all the other statistically demonstrated companions of arteriosclerosis. In our complex times such a single-minded approach to arteriosclerosis is not widely shared and is often derided as the false idol of the unsophisticated. Some respected professionals, however, support the worth of seeking a principal cause:

It has become something of a popular notion to say that the diseases we are left with, now that we have got rid of the major infections, are in some sense so complicated and so multifactorial, as the term goes—that they have something to do with the environment, or have something to do with stress and the pace of modern living. . . . I simply can't take that point of view very seriously—not as long as we are ignorant about the mechanisms of those diseases as we are. We really don't know anything at a deep level about the mechanism of heart disease, or cancer, or stroke or rheumatoid arthritis. We can make up stories about them, and it could be I suppose, that they have multiple causes, and are due to things we can't control in the environment. If that's true—if that should turn out to be true—that would be quite a piece of news. Because it has never happened before. Every disease that we do know about and for which we have really settled the issue, so that we can either turn it off, or prevent it once and for all—every such disease turns out to be a disease in which there is one central mechanism.

Lewis Thomas, M.D. (1978)
President, Memorial Sloan-Kettering Cancer Center

We present a theory of the origins of arteriosclerosis that has emerged from studies of dietary protein and vitamin B_6. The theory contradicts none of the familiar facts and observations, but explains them from a new perspective. It also suggests new measures of prevention and therapy.

The theory was first proposed in the medical literature by Dr. Kilmer McCully, professor of pathology at Harvard Medical School and Massachusetts General Hospital. It holds that high blood levels of homocysteine, a compound produced during digestion of protein, are central to the mechanism of arteriosclerosis. In addition, one can best understand the many observations concerning multiple risk factors by seeing how they affect homocysteine levels. Although the homocysteine theory itself is recent, the clinical and laboratory work supporting it has been carried out in a variety of places around the world over the last 70 years. The theory is based on a set of facts that have been tested and confirmed by medical researchers. They are the key pieces in the puzzle of arteriosclerosis and serve as a guide to the argument in our book:

- Arteriosclerosis is a slowly developing disease beginning early in life and continuing without symptoms for many years.
- Medical evidence suggests that this disease is primarily caused by environmental factors, particularly diet.
- People with a genetic disease called *homocystinuria* have a very high incidence of arteriosclerosis and begin to die of vascular problems in their first decade of life. They have high blood levels of homocysteine.
- Coronary patients have high residual levels of homocysteine in their blood.
- Healthy people generally have low amounts of homocysteine in their blood.
- Experimental animals given high regular doses of homocysteine rapidly develop arteriosclerosis. The intensity of the disease is directly related to the amounts of homocysteine the animals are given.
- Vitamin B_6 is required to clear homocysteine from the blood.

- People put on a diet low in vitamin B_6 for only a few weeks develop higher levels of homocysteine in their blood.
- Animals given a diet lacking vitamin B_6 develop humanlike arteriosclerosis. This occurs even in those animal species that tend to be resistant to cholesterol-induced arteriosclerosis.
- On the average, people who have had coronaries have much lower levels of vitamin B_6 in their blood than other people.
- In groups known to have chronic vitamin B_6 deficiencies, such as women taking birth control pills, deaths from cardiovascular disease are markedly increased over matched control groups.
- Because of the way we select, process, and cook foods, most people in the United States are only marginally supplied with vitamin B_6.

The pattern implicit in these facts is revealed by the homocysteine theory: *Arteriosclerosis is caused by homocysteine. Low levels of dietary vitamin B_6, in conjunction with high intake of protein, lead to toxic levels of homocysteine in the blood. Arteriosclerosis can be prevented or possibly reversed by reducing protein intake and insuring an adequate level of vitamin B_6.*

One of the real tests of a medical idea is whether or not it is clinically useful. The recommendations stemming from the homocysteine theory are not established practice and therefore the theory has not yet encountered this crucial test. On the other hand, the cholesterol hypothesis, long used as the basis for low-cholesterol dietary therapy, *has* been subjected to this test and has failed.

We decided to write a book on the homocysteine theory for two reasons: Like many physiologists, we have been surprised at the tenacious hold of the cholesterol hypothesis as an explanation of arteriosclerosis, given its poor success in guiding clinical treatment. Imagine if after the development of the Salk and Sabin polio vaccines there were almost as many cases of polio as before. The value of a fresh idea was obvious to us. Yet the more significant reason was our sense, which grew as we wrote the book, that the argument behind the homocysteine theory was more cohesive and comprehensive than could be guessed from the available literature. Part I of this book describes the nature of arteriosclerosis and the investigations that culminated in the homocysteine theory. The historical roots of the theory are embedded in the discoveries made mainly by scientists holding other points of view, including those favoring the cholesterol hypothesis. In Part II of the book, we use the homocysteine theory as a matrix for assessing diets and risk factors. We also consider how medical practices come to be accepted by physicians and their patients alike.

Part I
THE ROOTS OF
THE THEORY

CHAPTER 1
Arteriosclerosis

ARTERIOSCLEROSIS IS A WORLDWIDE EPIDEMIC. Victims have been diagnosed on every land mass on the planet. Yet not all populations are afflicted equally, and surveys showing the distribution of the disease provide intriguing clues into the ways diet and culture influence arteriosclerosis. Studying the incidence of a disease in populations of various environments is the task of the epidemiologist.

At the basis of epidemiological studies lies a more precise description of symptoms loosely covered by terms like "hardening of the arteries." A universal medical definition of the disease is valuable because it can then apply correctly and quantitatively whether the patient is from Liberia or Russia and appears vigorously healthy or nearly dead. So in order for us to refer unambiguously to the extent, location, and appearance of arteriosclerosis in both mildly and severely diseased arteries, we will give a medical description first of normal arteries and then of diseased ones. The description is not particularly complicated, but it may seem intimidating because it uses a medical vocabulary unfamiliar to many readers. We employ medical terms because they are precise and efficient and they convey an objective impression of the state of the arteries that is not tied to any particular interpretation or theory of causation. Armed with this background, we will find our later encounters with epidemiology, clinical reports, and experimental studies more fruitful than if we merely made do with the vague images most of us have of where arteriosclerosis happens, how much change it represents, and what those changes look like. The

3

reader will gain deeper perspective by reading the next sections (especially when we refer to particular studies), but you can read much of the book profitably without this material. Thus, if you prefer, you can begin the text with the description of clinical symptoms on page 11.

THE NORMAL ARTERY

The wall of a healthy artery is smooth and pliable. It feels like a half-cooked noodle. The hollow of the vessel is called the

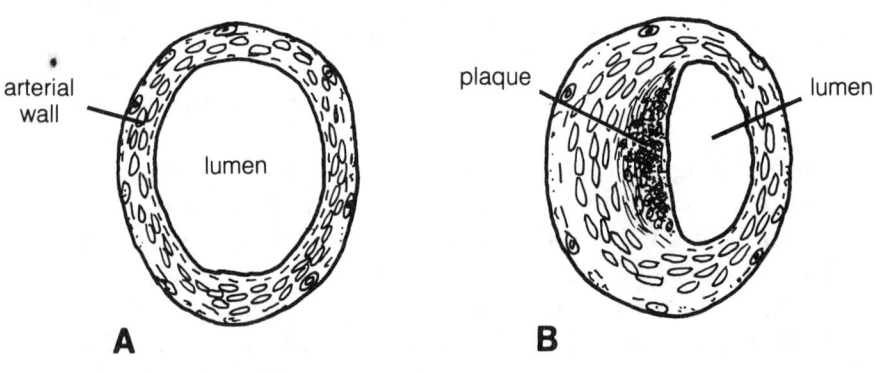

These drawings show cross-sections of normal (A) and diseased (B) arteries. The hollow central area where blood flows is called the lumen. In diseased arteries plaques build up in the arterial wall. This has the effect of narrowing the lumen; as a result, less blood flows through the artery.

lumen. In a normal artery, the lumen is completely open to the flow of blood.

The arterial wall consists of three layers. Only the innermost layer, the *intima*, is normally in direct, or *intimate*, contact with the blood coursing through the vessel. The intima is lined with a sheet of flattened cells called *endothelial* cells. This lining is so thin that the endothelial cells do not pile up, but instead lie adjacent to each other, touching at their edges to form a layer only one cell thick. Outside the endothelial lining is a tough grid of elastic fibers called the *internal elastic lamina*.

Blood flows fast and nonturbulently wherever the intima is smooth and unpuckered. With age, the intimal layer grows thicker and some cells from the second layer of the arterial wall, the *media*, can be found in it. The media contains smooth muscle, which contracts the artery and counters the stretching produced by increases in local blood pressure. Smooth muscles are so called because of their smooth appearance under the microscope and are distinguished from the striated muscles we use in moving around. As you can see in the drawing on the next page, the media is much thicker than the intima.

The outermost layer of the vessel wall, the *adventitia*, is separated from the media by a second grid of elastic fibers similar to the one that separates the media from the intima, but which is thinner and looser. The adventitia consists of a loosely packed mix of cells, fibrous protein, and other molecules. Nerves, capillaries, and small blood vessels supplying the cells of the arterial wall are also found in the adventitia.

DISEASED ARTERIES

As the arterial wall becomes diseased, the most obvious change is that it becomes harder and thicker. It seems natural therefore to refer to the disease as *arteriosclerosis* ("artery" plus *sclerosis*, which means "hardening"). The most common form of arteriosclerosis is *atherosclerosis*. The first signs of atherosclerosis appear when the internal elastic lamina frays, allowing smooth muscle cells of the media to migrate inward to the intima. These muscle cells aggregate, and connective tissue

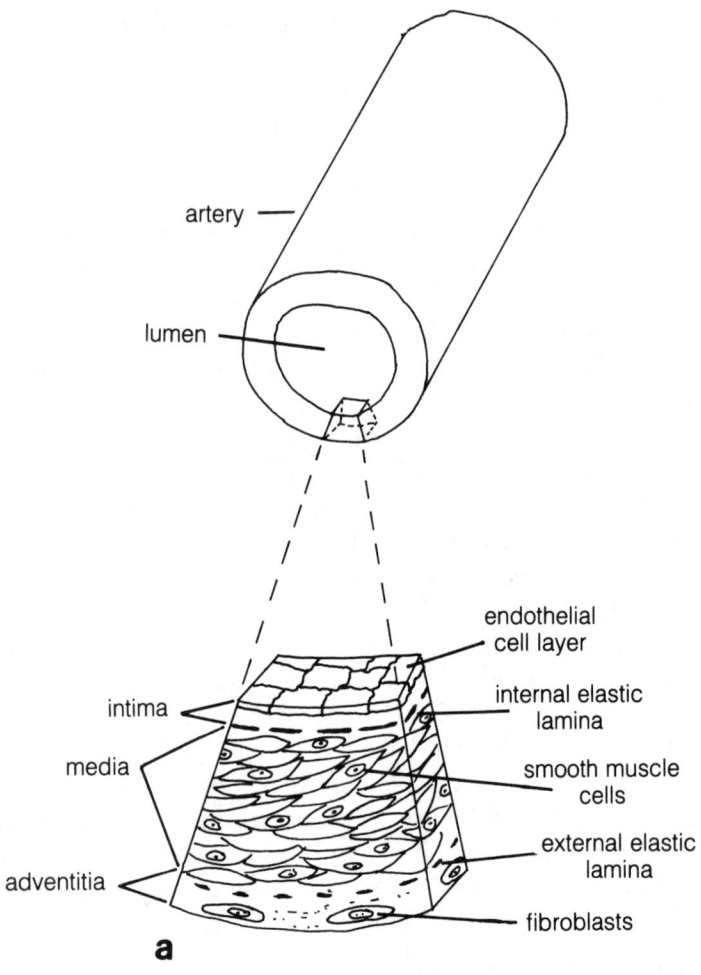

artery

lumen

endothelial
cell layer

intima

internal elastic
lamina

media

smooth muscle
cells

external elastic
lamina

adventitia

fibroblasts

a

(a) normal arterial wall
(b) – (d) changes in the arterial wall as arteriosclerosis
develops. The endothelial layer is stripped away in patches,
while smooth muscle cells from the media invade the intima
through the frayed internal elastic lamina. The plaque grows
into the lumen, calcifying and taking up fats. It becomes a site
for clot (thrombus) formation (after Ross and Glomset 1976).

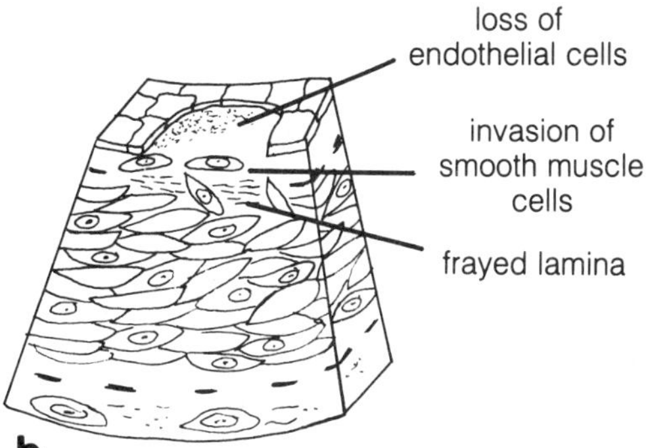

loss of
endothelial cells

invasion of
smooth muscle
cells

frayed lamina

b

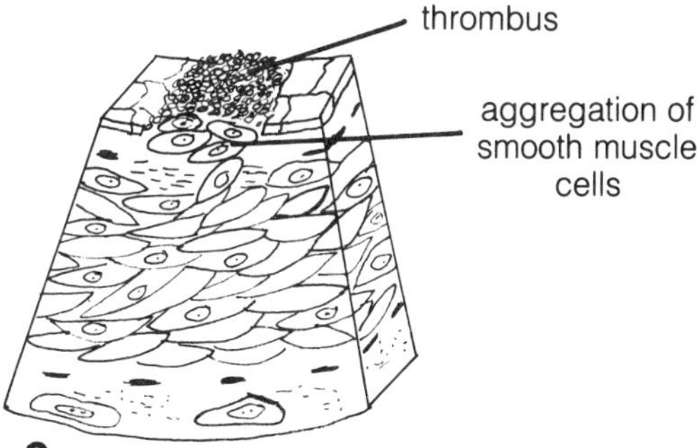

thrombus

aggregation of
smooth muscle
cells

c

complicated
lesion

d

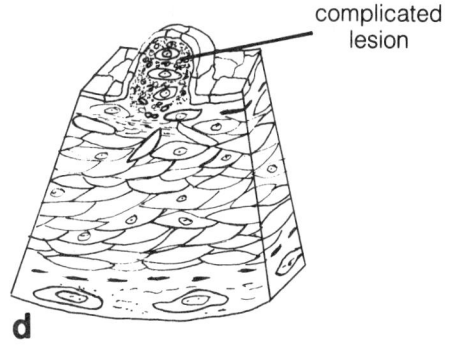

forms around them. The resulting mass contains at this point little or no cholesterol or related fats. Decades ago, investigators thought this *fibromusculoelastic lesion* arose after a deposition of cholesterol from the blood. However, anatomical studies have since shown that the migration of muscle cells is the initial structural sign of *plaque* formation.

The plaque alters with time, and cholesterol and fat do eventually accumulate, forming an *atheroma*. At first, the atheroma appears white and it is just large enough to protrude into the lumen. With time the atheroma grows larger, as muscle cells proliferate and lipids (fats) and other substances accumulate. The plaque is now an advanced or "complicated" lesion. As the plaque thickens, the arterial wall is distorted out of round, and calcium from the blood stream begins to deposit in the plaque. Calcium binds to proteins and other substances, causing the wall to harden. The atheroma expands into the lumen, sometimes to the point of blocking, or occluding, the artery. The narrowed regions of arteries greatly increase the hazard represented by clots (thromboses), which tend to form at atheromas. Clots that circulate can lodge in narrowed channels and block the flow of blood. In badly diseased vessels, atheromas can cover more than 50 percent of the surface area of the wall. Blood flow is often turbulent; since the arterial wall is no longer elastic, its ability to exert a smoothing effect is vastly reduced. In fact, *calcification* can become so pronounced that one can hear crackling as the arteries are bent.

In American adults the inner surface of the aorta is frequently covered with sharp-edged, hard protuberances, which feel like broken bits of glass embedded in the wall. At autopsy pathologists routinely cut the aorta open along its length, and the crunching sound made by the scissors as they encounter the calcified regions is quite prominent. The wall of the aorta may be grossly distorted with bumps and pebbly ridges, which induce local twists and bendings along the whole surface. No microscope is needed to detect the sort of pathology common to the large arteries of most adults.

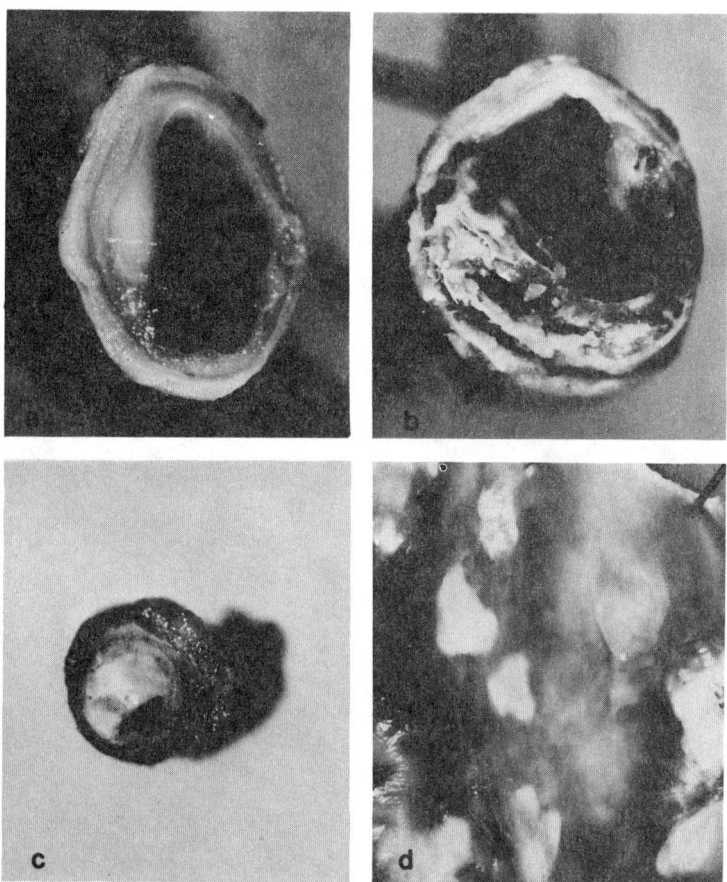

Examples of arteriosclerosis. These photographs show different arteries obtained from a 59-year-old man who had died in 1979 of an acute coronary attack several hours before autopsy. The severity of the arteriosclerosis varies. In (a), (b), and (c) the vessels were cut crosswise with a sharp scalpel and viewed end on. (a) Femoral artery. An atheroma, on the left, is beginning to encroach into the lumen. (b) Iliac artery. This lesion is more advanced and the plaque has already calcified and hardened. Sharp pieces broken off by the cutting of the artery can be seen. (c) Left coronary artery. The lumen is almost completely filled in. (d) Inner surface of the aorta. The white patches are individual plaques. Compare (d) with the illustration on p. 15 of the aorta of Dr. Wepfer, who died in 1695, which shows similar patches.

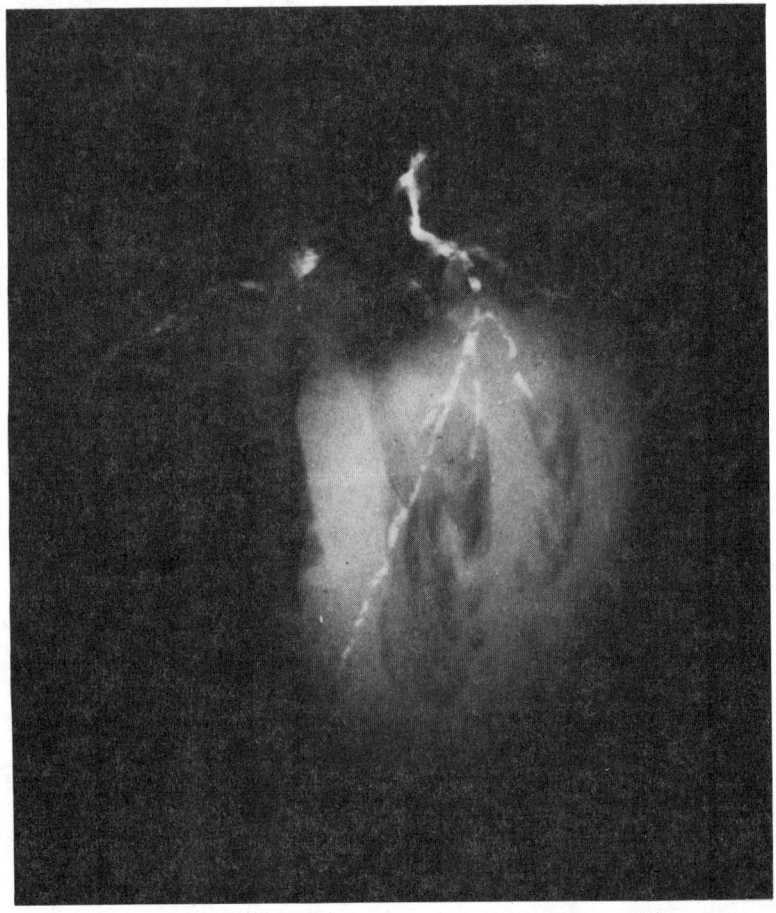

X-ray negative of a heart: The coronary arteries supplying the heart muscle envelope the heart in a vascular network. They are normally invisible in X-ray photographs since arteries are soft tissue and produce no contrast with the tissue of the heart. In this patient, however, the coronary arteries are so calcified that they stand out as an array of branches extending down over the heart. The patchy character of the branches reflects local variation of the severity of arteriosclerosis. This patient has unusually advanced arteriosclerosis.

ATHEROSCLEROSIS AND ARTERIOSCLEROSIS

Although theories explaining plaque initiation have changed through the years, the observations of the structural pathology of the vessels we have just outlined have remained consistent for decades. Unfortunately, the names for the disease have been used with much less consistency and they now frequently create confusion. In 1904 Dr. Felix Marchand introduced "atherosclerosis" as the name for the disease characterized by lesions of progressive severity in the arterial walls culminating in atheromas. Because it explicitly refers to the most frequently observed progression of arterial wall disease, it is preferred by many medical authors.

"Arteriosclerosis," on the other hand, refers to hardening of the arteries produced by any disease conditions. Its first use in 1833 is entirely consistent with contemporary use. Despite the reservations of some physicians who consider "arteriosclerosis" too vague, there are no signs of the term disappearing from the medical literature. Indeed, some authors use arteriosclerosis and atherosclerosis interchangeably. We will use arteriosclerosis to refer to the general problem of sclerotic vascular disease, and atherosclerosis to refer to the well-studied form of the disease most frequently encountered in clinical pathology.

CLINICAL SYMPTOMS

When an atheroma expands to the extent of occluding an artery, blood cannot flow past the block, and tissue beyond the atheroma dies from lack of oxygen. Atheromas occur often in branches of the coronary arteries that supply the heart muscle cells. They may block off a branch so extensively as to kill the part of the heart served by that branch. This is a *myocardial infarction,* or heart attack. When a brain artery is suddenly occluded, a stroke results.

Arteriosclerotic arteries are more likely to block than normal arteries. The condition is systemic, potentially affecting any organ in the body, but the heart and brain are most vulnerable because their cells are served primarily by only one arterial branch. Other tissues, such as skin and muscle, have collateral circulation, which takes over if blocks occur.

If the disease impedes the flow of blood in coronary arteries without blocking them completely, *angina pectoris* may result. This pain in the chest or arms can vary from noticeable to incapacitating and is made more intense by exercise or work. Although many angina sufferers are able to remain active at their jobs, others must be confined to bed.

Similar disease in the arterial supply to the kidney can produce an elevation in blood pressure, which increases hazards of *aneurysm* (ballooning of vessels) and bursting of blood vessels. The kidney produces a hormone, called renin, that through activation of another molecule, angiotensin, influences blood pressure. Arteriosclerosis in the renal (kidney) artery leads to a restriction of blood supply to the kidney. The kidney reacts as though blood pressure were too low and increases the level of angiotensin. Blood pressure rises until the flow of blood is restored. As arteriosclerosis worsens and the blood flow becomes more restricted, more angiotensin is produced and *hypertension* (high blood pressure) results. This is one of the ways arteriosclerosis creates high blood pressure.

Taken together, vascular diseases account for about half of the deaths in the United States each year. Heart disease and cerebrovascular disease are also listed as major causes of death in all other developed countries.

NATURAL HISTORY OF ARTERIOSCLEROSIS

At this point, several questions arise. Is arteriosclerosis new? Did it first appear in humans with the invention of the wheel, the aqueduct, or the steam engine? Or, is it an older plague, possibly shared with other animal species descended from the same arteriosclerotic ancestors? Another important question concerns the geographical distribution of the disease. What are the clues one can legitimately extract from epidemiology and what are the limitations? Are there any contemporary human cultures that are symptom free?

No fossils of blood vessels of our evolutionary ancestors are sufficiently preserved for study of the extent of arteriosclerosis. Soft tissues are prone to decay and survive for only a short time except in a few rare cases—the woolly mammoths that became frozen in the glacial ice sheets of Siberia, for example, or the itinerant hags and barbarians that were entrapped and then preserved in the peat bogs of northern Europe. To our knowledge their blood vessels have not been studied.

Another form of preservation has been artificial. In some cultures men embalmed a few of their citizens and the record of arteriosclerotic specimens over the last 5,000 years is surprisingly good as a consequence. By the XVIII Dynasty of King Tutankhamen and Queen Hatshepsut, Egyptian embalmers had developed sufficient skill that even after 3,000 years muscles and skin have not rotted. Unfortunately, however, in order to keep the amount of soft tissue to a minimum, the heart and major blood vessels were usually discarded with the entrails. In 1910, Marc Ruffer, an English physician working in Cairo, investigated the arteries of several mummies. Usually the muscles of the arms were removed along with those of the rest of the body, and the resulting holes were stuffed with mud, sand, and rags. However, sometimes the limbs escaped this part of the process (because, as Ruffer suggested, "the embalmers had evidently scamped their work") and on these occasions they were preserved intact. Ruffer (1910) found a generous amount of arteriosclerosis in the large arteries of these limbs.

There can be no doubt respecting the calcification of the arteries, and that it is exactly of the same nature as we see at the present day, namely, calcification following on atheroma. The small patches seen in the arteries are atheromatous, and though the vessels have without doubt been altered by the 3000 years or so which have elapsed since death, nevertheless the lesions are still recognizable by their position and microscopic structure. . . . The disease is characterized by a marked degeneration of the muscular coat and of the endothelium. These diseased patches, discrete at first, fuse together later, and finally form comparatively large areas of degenerated tissue, which may reach the

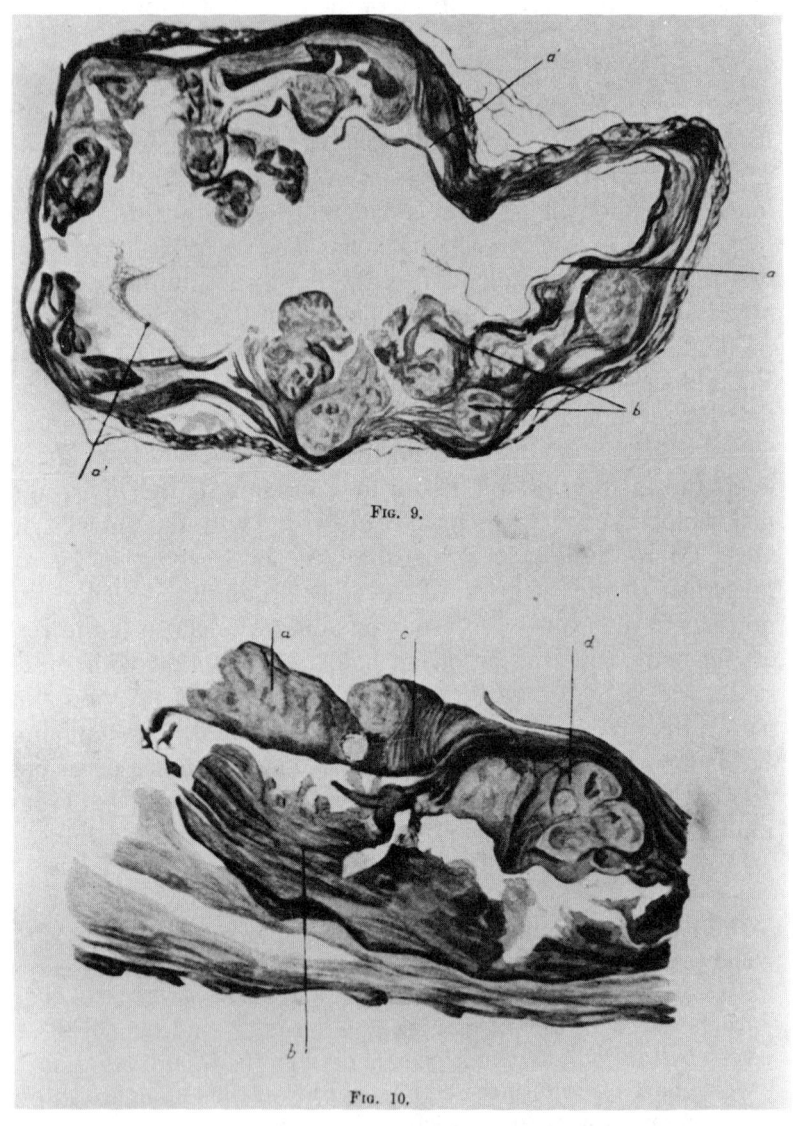

Fig. 9.

Fig. 10.

Lithograph of arteriosclerotic arteries of ancient Egyptian mummies (from Ruffer 1910). Calcified patches are pointed out by the author (b and d).

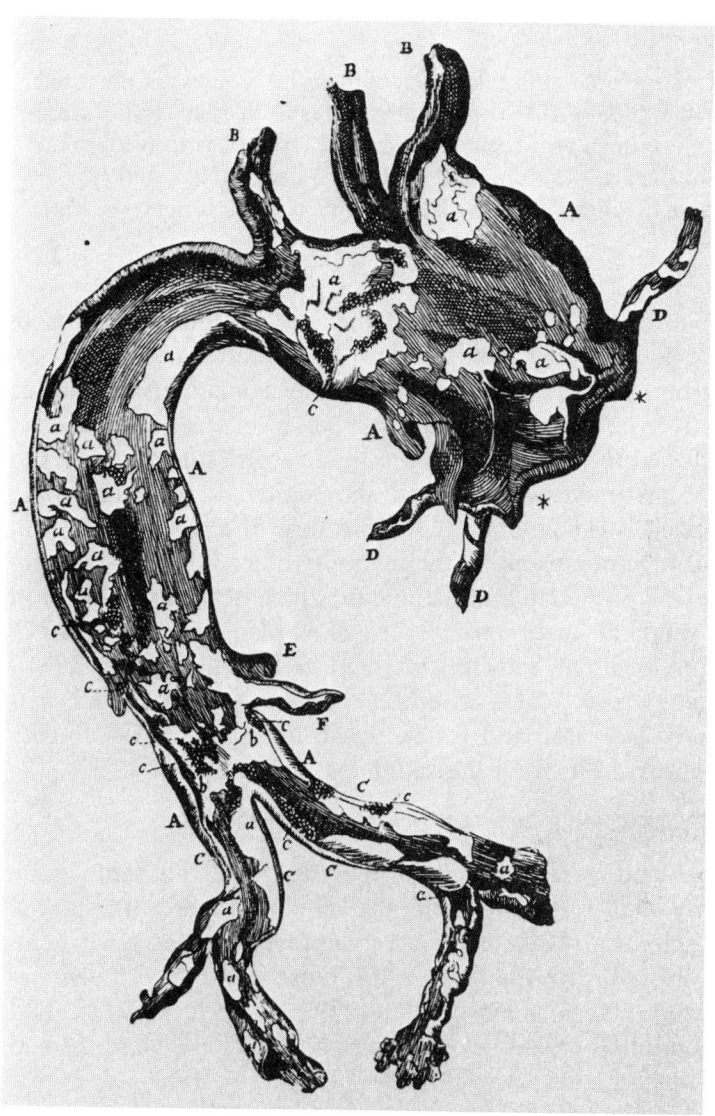

A woodcut of the aorta of the physician Johann Jakob Wepfer drawn in 1695. It was first published in 1727. The aorta has been opened up along its length and the inside surface is visible. Areas marked by *a* represent plaques. Compare the distribution of plaques with those from a recent specimen (photograph d on page 9).

surface and open into the lumen of the tube. I need not point out how completely this description agrees with that of the same disease as seen at the present time. . . . When we consider that few of the arteries examined were quite healthy, it would appear that such lesions were as frequent 3000 years ago as they are today.

Ancient Egyptians were not the only historical victims of arteriosclerosis, and clear medical descriptions of the disease date from the time of the first modern anatomist, Vesalius (1514–1564). These became part of a clinical record that stretches to the present. Such a long record suggests that the disease has been common and shows that early practitioners recognized it as a pathology. For instance, the physician Johann Conrad Brunner attended the necropsy of his father-in-law, the pioneering physician and pathologist, Johann Jakob Wepfer, in 1695. Wepfer's aorta contained calcified plaques so hard that at the time Brunner referred to them as bonelike (Long 1967). Brunner wrote, "The internal coat in several places was ruptured, lacerated and rotten like fruit, and hurt the fingers when thrust in it, from the roughness of the bones."

ARTERIOSCLEROSIS IN ANIMALS

The blood vessels of all vertebrates have the same basic anatomy. So it is not surprising that all vertebrates show signs of arteriosclerosis. Humans are not unique. Studies have been done on both wild animals and those that have been sequestered in zoos. Forty years ago, Dr. H. Fox (1933) studied 10,000 animals from the Philadelphia Zoological Garden, and more recently Dr. R. Finlayson (1965), a pathologist at the Royal College of Surgeons, has examined 1,500 specimens at the London Zoological Gardens. Compared to man, all other vertebrates have less severe arteriosclerosis. Yet animals that live in man-made environments in zoos and eat diets selected by humans show greater arteriosclerosis than do animals in the wild.

Arteriosclerosis is slight in both carnivorous mammals (tigers, leopards, dogs) that eat mostly meat and herbivorous mammals (elephants, rabbits, deer) that eat vegetarian diets low in saturated fats. Birds and primates have more pronounced arteriosclerosis than other vertebrates, such as reptiles, amphibians, and fish, where the disease occurs only rarely. The severity of arteriosclerosis is not constant even for individuals within a species. In Pacific salmon, for example, a sudden and rapid increase in arteriosclerosis occurs during the migration associated with spawning. Salmon caught in the ocean are essentially free of the disease (Robertson et al. 1961). However, during their migration to freshwater breeding pools, the fish suffer progressive vascular deterioration. After spawning, the fishes' hearts and blood vessels show extensive calcification and arteriosclerosis. Such vascular changes are the primary factors in death, which usually occurs soon after spawning.

The relation between blood pressure and the presence of arteriosclerosis is obscure and evidence from animals does little to clarify it. In man, the mortal risk of high blood pressure is well established; vessels like the pulmonary artery, which have relatively lower pressure than other arteries in the body, are also consistently freer of arteriosclerosis. Giraffes, however, have very high blood pressure at the level of the heart in order to push the column of blood up their long necks. Yet they show little arteriosclerosis.

In animals, as in humans, arteriosclerosis worsens with age: older animals show both more severe disease and higher incidence of disease than younger animals of the same species. This holds equally for animals in the laboratory or in the wild. In laboratory environments, experimenters can feed diets that produce severe arteriosclerosis in species that are susceptible. Herbivorous rabbits, for example, are rarely affected by arteriosclerosis in the wild, but they have become the classic animals for experimental studies as a result of their susceptibility on laboratory diets. The disease has also been induced in omnivorous animals such as monkeys, but with greater effort. It is exceedingly difficult to induce the disease in carnivorous animals such as dogs and cats.

DISTRIBUTION OF ARTERIOSCLEROSIS

It is well known that older people have arteriosclerosis, but so do younger people who do not exhibit any obvious symptoms. During the Korean War a large-scale study was carried out on young U.S. soldiers killed accidentally or in combat. Dr. William Enos and his colleagues (1953) at the Armed Forces Institute of Pathology in Washington, D.C., performed autopsies on 300 such casualties.

These soldiers had been in good general health, had successfully gone through the rigors of basic training, and had normal blood pressure. The coronary arteries were subjected to microscopic examination for assessment of the degree of arteriosclerosis. Although the average age of the 300 soldiers, 22.1 years, was far younger than that commonly associated with heart attack or stroke, the results obtained upset any comfortable security in the belief that young people are free of "hardened arteries." Fully 77 percent showed "gross evidence of coronary arteriosclerosis." The clinical severity ranged from fibrous plaques to complete occlusion of the coronary arteries. In 14 cases more than one of the main branches of the coronary artery was at least 80 percent occluded by widespread arteriosclerotic lesions.

Other studies on groups of young, apparently healthy, men without previous history of heart disease confirm that arteriosclerosis is widespread among the young.

In 1963 Dr. J.K. Mason of the Royal Air Force Institute of Pathology in England reported that of 275 healthy young men who had died in accidents, 21.8 percent had atherosclerotic restrictions of coronary arteries and 34.5 percent had macroscopic (visible to the naked eye) atherosclerotic coronary disease. More recently (1971), Dr. J.J. McNamara and his U.S. Army colleagues found that among combat casualties in Vietnam, again, average age 22.1 years, "45 percent of young healthy American males had some degree of atherosclerosis." In fact, the conclusion that young people have extensive arteriosclerosis had been reported years earlier. Dr. J.G. Monkeberg studied German soldier casualties in World War I. Coronary arteriosclerosis was found in 353 of the 652 autopsies he carried out.

The results of the investigations of war casualties show that although arteriosclerosis is infamous for debilitating or killing older people, ostensibly normal, healthy people in their twenties also have the disease.

ARTERIOSCLEROSIS IN INFANTS

Even younger people are afflicted. A number of studies have been made of the extent of arteriosclerosis in infants that have died from various illnesses and accidents. One of the most convincing and extensive surveys was performed by Dr. Doris Jaffe and her colleagues at the Research Institute of the Hospital for Sick Children in Toronto and published in 1971. Working from a sample of 176 infants who had died in their first month after birth, Jaffe and the others examined the babies' hearts and arteries under the microscope. The team, like others who had carried out similar studies, noticed "cushions," or thickening, of the intima. The thickenings tended to occur at points where the coronary arteries branched and they varied in degree from negligible to so massive that they seriously compromised blood flow and were considered to be the possible cause of death. "Normal" arteries were extremely rare. Only six of the 157 specimens catalogued for degree of thickening were free of the disease, having an endothelial layer lying directly on a smooth, intact internal elastic lamina. Most of the specimens showed intimal thickenings consisting of a proliferation of both cells and fibers within the intima. Also, the internal elastic lamina was fragmented and it appeared that smooth muscle cells had passed through it into the intima. As we pointed out earlier, such lesions constitute the first stage of atherosclerosis. Yet since virtually every infant had some intimal thickening, Jaffe and her colleagues were hesitant to conclude that these thickenings were abnormal.

Regardless of the reason for the formation of branch site thickenings, their regular presence so early in life suggests that they are normal anatomical structures. And yet, the massive bulk in some cases is surely indicative of some pathological process. We conclude that coronary branch sites in the newborn infant are normally provided with musculoelastic pads which are prone to undergo a pathological overgrowth.

However, since there was no obvious demarcation to show the boundary between normal branch pads and pathological thickening of the intima, the authors described a "continuous range," suggesting that even the fatal cases were not "examples of a rare disorder, but, rather, extreme examples of a common condition." The report was extremely cautious and refrained from any direct diagnosis of atherosclerosis. It emphasized, instead, the continuity of the observed pads and later sites of atherosclerotic disease (other groups have reported similar observations). Jaffe and her collaborators also argued that since the intima was often quite severely thickened at birth, "antenatal factors" of some unknown kind must play an important part in determining the condition of the walls of blood vessels even before birth.

So, pathology reveals that arteriosclerosis, common at all ages, is severe in old people, less severe in adults, and has its antecedents in infants and, at least by inference, in fetuses. Furthermore, studies from other Western countries agree with these findings. The pervasiveness of arteriosclerosis appears to be so general that every man, woman, and child throughout most of the world is to some extent a victim of the disease. This is particularly true for North Americans and Western Europeans.

One of the significant consequences of this ubiquity of arteriosclerosis is that any exceptions become extremely interesting. Are there any counterexamples, people who prove, by being relatively free of arteriosclerosis themselves, that it is possible for humans to live on this planet, eat its food and water, and yet have elastic, healthy arteries with a minimum of "intimal thickenings"?

EXCEPTIONS

On the basis of observations made in modern Israel, the answer seems to be yes. Several epidemiological studies have been conducted in Israel because its diverse ethnic groups have quite different rates of heart disease. Many Israelis are Ashkenazi Jews who have emigrated from Europe. They suffer an extremely high rate of heart disease. Another important group, Yemenite Jews, who emigrated from Asia Minor, have a generally lower rate than the Ashkenazim.

A third population, the object of our quest for an exception to the universality of arteriosclerosis, consists of Bedouin Moslems, who have one of the lowest rates of heart attack in the world. In comparison with the cosmopolitan Ashkenazim who live in cities and on modern kibbutzim, the Bedouins live a very different kind of life. Epidemiologists have tried to discover some quality in the nature of the Bedouins' environment to account for the difference in vascular disease.

The Bedouins live in the Negev, a triangular wedge of land, which makes up southern Israel. The area is usually considered a desert since much of it is desolate and rugged. It is dominated by a high, dry plateau and contains occasional sand dunes. But in the winter months, parts of the Negev receive marginal rainfall, approximately as much as falls on the region of the American Great Plains on the eastern edge of the Rocky Mountains. There are 20,000 *Badawi* (Arabic for "desert dweller"), or Bedouins, who inhabit the area. They are seminomadic. They grow wheat and barley on the parsimonious clay soil and graze sheep, goats, cows, and camels on wild pastureland. The young boys and girls and the married women shepherd the flocks while others tend the fields (Groen et al. 1964).

In 1969 Dr. Z. Vlodaver and Dr. H. N. Neufeld from the Heart Institute of the University of Tel-Aviv Medical School and Dr. Harold Kahn of the National Heart Institute in Bethesda, Maryland, published a report on the coronary arteries of Ashkenazi Jews, Yemenite Jews, and Bedouins. They examined fetuses, infants, and children younger than ten years. All had died of accident or infection. Working with many slices cut from 211 coronary arteries, the investigators measured the cross-sectional areas of the innermost layers of the arterial walls. The results showed that Bedouins had very thin arterial walls in comparison to the Ashkenazi and Yemenite Jews. Furthermore, the difference in intimal thickening became greater with increasing age. The Bedouin children retained thin intimal layers, whereas the Ashkenazi children, particularly the males, showed progressive thickening of the walls. Bedouins had what could be displayed as textbook examples of normal healthy coronary arteries with a single layer of endothelium in the intima and no invasion by smooth muscle cells. The intima thickened slightly with age, but much less steeply than that of Yemenites or Ashkenazi Jews. These results clearly indicate that a thickened intima is not a universal phenomenon in young children.

Dr. Vlodaver and his co-workers had been motivated to pursue their study by the low incidence of clinical atherosclerosis among adult Bedouins. Heart attacks are so rare that another group studying 510 men, all over the age of 30, found only one case of heart trouble, and he was 70 years old (Groen et al. 1964).

Although Bedouins have been the most extensively studied examples of exceptional cardiovascular health, reports indicate that nomads in the arctic once had very little heart disease as well. Physicians serving 40 to 50 years ago as medical officers for expeditions to Northern Labrador, Greenland, and northern Canada wrote striking descriptions of the cardiovascular health of Eskimo populations not heavily exposed to Western civilization (Thomas 1927). In 1936 Dr. I.M. Rabinowitch, a Canadian physician engaged to perform field studies in the arctic, undertook physical examinations (which included measurements of blood pressure) of several hundred people living as far south as Hudson Bay and as far north as northern Baffin Island. Baffin Island Eskimos, who lived and hunted as their ancestors had before contact with white traders or missionaries, had "no

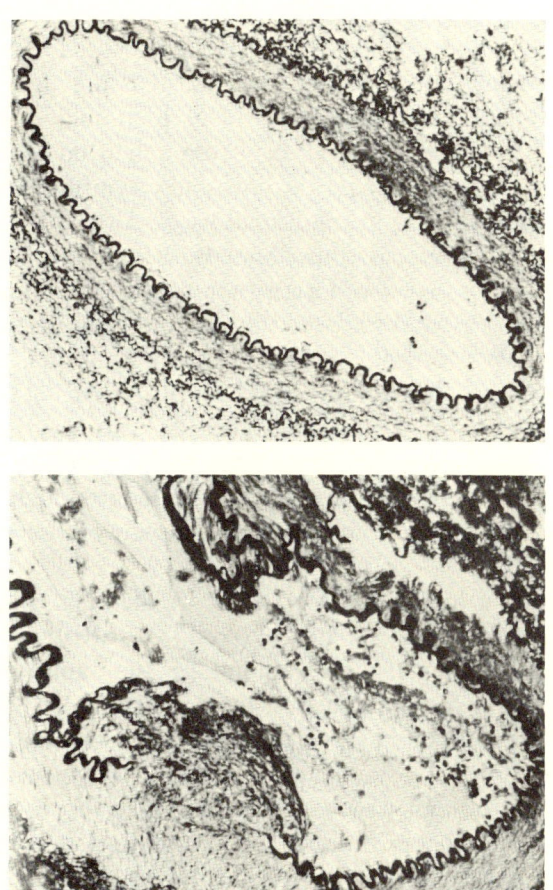

(top) Artery of a young Bedouin female. The artery was cut in cross-section, and is a textbook-like example of a healthy looking artery. The internal elastic lamina is intact and appears as a dark scalloped line on the inner border. In life, the pressure of the blood within would stretch the wall, and the internal elastic lamina would be smooth. The endothelial layer is too thin to be seen at this magnification, but is normal (from Vlodaver et al. 1969 by permission of the American Heart Association, Inc.). (bottom) Artery from a patient with arteriosclerosis, similarly prepared. Note the fraying of the internal elastic lamina at the thickenings (from McCully 1969 by permission of Dr. McCully).

arteriosclerosis." In contrast, the more assimilated Eskimos around Hudson Bay had a relatively high incidence of the disease. Other physicians, all of whom relied on their clinical observations, have reported cardiovascular symptoms to be rare among Eskimos living in traditional ways. Although anatomical investigations, such as those on the Bedouins, were not performed, later Alaskan autopsy studies have confirmed that arteriosclerosis is quite low in the Eskimo population. A 1960 report by A.W. Gottman of 57 Eskimos and Aleuts, for example, uncovered a death rate due to arteriosclerosis of 6 percent, a figure about one-tenth the Caucasian rate in the United States. The difference in death rate can not be attributed to the possibility that Eskimos do not live long enough to die of heart attack or stroke: many of the 57 cases were over 50 years of age.

In a parallel autopsy report by B. Arthaud in 1970 of 250 cases, 10 percent of the deaths could be attributed to cardiovascular problems. And remember, the samples in both studies were of necessity biased toward populations who were close to medical personnel and thus tending to lead less traditional lives. It seems reasonable to suppose that cardiovascular problems were even rarer among more "primitive" Eskimos. In 1972 S.A. Feldman and a team visited the Tigara Eskimos of the North Slope of Alaska, who still lived by hunting whales from hide-covered boats. This team stated that these Eskimos "develop atherosclerosis mild in degree, of limited clinical significance, and certainly did not account for one of the major causes of death among them."

Interestingly, arteriosclerosis is not the only disease affected by contact with traders and missionaries. Other regional differences, for example in tooth decay, were found by Rabinowitch (1936) to be correlated with Western influence, in this case, with the practice of tooth brushing.

Groups of people relatively free from arteriosclerosis are rare, and as such are extremely important as sources for inquiry into the key environmental factor or factors that set them apart. We should mention two more groups. In 1974 Dr. P.F. Sinnett and

Dr. H.M. Whyte of the University of Papua, New Guinea, studied a highland population in Tukisenta. They reported that ischemic heart disease (caused by compromised blood flow through the coronary arteries) is "rare if not absent" among these people. In addition, in contrast to Western populations, this highland population does not show increased blood pressure and serum cholesterol with age.

The second group comes to our notice through the recollections of an Egyptian physician, Abd El-Aziz Ismail, of Cairo. Dr. Ismail had both a private and a charity practice beginning about 1913. In 1928 he wrote that although 10 percent of the cases in his private practice concerned chronic hypertension, his charity patients, who were very poor, never exhibited high blood pressure. In fact, in all 15 years of treating several thousand charity patients, he could count only two genuine hypertensives. Ismail did not directly measure the incidence of arteriosclerosis for these poor patients, but he suggested that the group was uniquely resistant to the disease.

ENVIRONMENTAL FACTORS

Do these groups have little arteriosclerosis and arteriosclerotic heart disease because they are genetically unique or because their diet, behavior, or some other aspect of their culture prevents the disease? Bedouins subsist mainly on rarif, a cooked bread made from crudely milled whole wheat flour. They eat meat on the average of once a month, and have a particularly low dietary intake of cholesterol. They show no vitamin deficiencies.

Eskimos, on the other hand, follow a completely different diet. In fact, the word *Eskimo* derives from the language of the Cree Indians, who called these arctic nomads *Uskipoo:* "he eats raw meat," a practice the Cree found offensive (Sinclair 1953). The traditional Eskimo diet consisted almost entirely of large amounts of raw meat and fish. This diet was very low in carbohydrates, but by worldwide comparison, contained astonishing quantities of protein and animal fat. Sinclair observed that when food was plentiful, the Eskimos would commonly eat about nine pounds of meat daily. Traditional Eskimos, like the Bedouins, showed no vitamin deficiencies.

Low incidence of arteriosclerosis is the common feature of the Bedouin, Arctic, and New Guinea studies. This observation does not by itself provide a clue as to whether the low rate of arteriosclerosis can be explained on the basis of genetic or environmental factors. Using epidemiological methods, it is possible to assess the importance of environmental factors such as diet, but not by means of the sort of study we have considered so far. And until that question is settled it is not possible to tell if studying the Bedouin, Eskimo, or Tukisenta can suggest ways for curing the rest of us. They may be the lucky beneficiaries of a much restricted genetic mix rather than practitioners of some cultural pattern we could emulate. Although the evidence that Western culture influences the incidence of arteriosclerosis in Eskimos suggests environmental factors, further evidence is needed.

One way to measure the impact of environmental factors on incidence of arteriosclerosis is to monitor a particular ethnic group in different settings. For instance, Dr. M. Toor and a group of colleagues in Israel (1960) studied the change in the "atherosclerotic mortality rate" for Yemenite immigrants to Israel. They compared "early Yemenites," people from Yemen who had lived in Israel for more than 20 years, with "recent Yemenites," people who had lived in Israel for about five years. Both groups were considered to have been of the same genetic stock.

Toor and his colleagues found that "early" male Yemenites had four times the rate of atherosclerotic mortality of "recent" male Yemenites (they were all in the 45–60 age group). "Early" female Yemenites had three times the rate of "recent" female Yemenites. Yet the mortality from other diseases was the same for both groups. Thus, among populations of the same age, those who had lived the longest in Israel had a much higher incidence of arteriosclerosis than recent arrivals. A major dietary difference between the two groups was that "early" Yemenites ate more fats and protein than "recent" arrivals.

These results suggest that environmental factors are indeed important.

The Toor study is consistent with similar studies on other populations. The epidemiologist Dr. Ancel Keys and his colleagues in Minnesota and Japan (1958) compared the extent of arteriosclerosis in Japanese living in Japan with that of the Japanese living in Hawaii and the mainland of the United States. They performed autopsies on Japanese between ages 50 and 69 who had died in Japan and Hawaii, regardless of cause of death. Keys found "severe arteriosclerosis" in approximately 10 percent of the Japan-dwelling Japanese and in approximately 30 percent of the Japanese living in Hawaii. The team further asserted that the rate of severe arteriosclerosis reached 70 percent for Japanese in the U.S. mainland (though this contention was not supported by direct evidence from pathological examinations). Unless one can envision some consistent underlying genetic variation, which Keys considered unlikely, such differences must be accounted for by variation in environment and culture in each locality.

STATIONARY POPULATIONS

For stationary populations, the extent of the environmental influences on arteriosclerosis can be tested if conditions change so as to affect the entire population. During World War II military blockades or occupations disrupted conditions in many countries so that diet and other aspects of daily life changed drastically. Finland, for example, was attacked by Russia and was isolated from shipments of food. Norway and the Netherlands were occupied by Germany. The rate of heart attacks plummeted in these countries. For instance, in Finland in 1940, 1,720 people died of arteriosclerosis (Vartiainen and Kanerva 1947). By 1943 only 540 people died of arteriosclerosis (in 1941 and 1942 the figures were 1,510 and 1,020, respectively). Considering the presumed level of stress, the reduction in arteriosclerosis is surprising. As Ancel Keys (1975) remarks, "A major lesson gained from World War II is the proof that in a very few years the incidence of coronary heart disease could drop to a level on the order of one-fourth the preceding rate."

Equally significant, after the war the incidence of coronary heart disease in these countries climbed back to prewar levels within a short period. By contemporary standards, the drop and rise were both enormous. The large-scale drop proves that arteriosclerosis, though epidemic, is not immutable and can be reduced substantially in whole populations by some environmental changes. Which features of the environment are crucial remain a substantial mystery. Although we have not yet suggested what Bedouins and Eskimos do right, the results of the epidemiological studies in Europe indicate that they *do* something, and don't just sit on their genes. We could expect that if an infant Ashkenazi Jew were to be adopted by a nomadic Bedouin family, he would develop less arteriosclerosis than if he were to remain in his original cultural environment.

What could Israeli Bedouins, poor Egyptians in the 1920s, wilderness Eskimos, and highland New Guineans have in common that would also be shared, but only transiently, by beleaguered Dutchmen and Finns? And why does arteriosclerosis tend to worsen with age? That fact has been with us so long that it is almost taken for granted, even though many other diseases do not show the same relation to age.

Epidemiological studies have limitations that make it hard to resolve such questions with certainty. Skeptics can point to sampling problems. For instance, people who collect data must perforce have at least slightly different criteria. The population under study may have a hidden bias. For example, poor people might never visit a clinic for a symptom, such as chest pain, that would impel rich people to consult their physicians immediately. Or, the criteria for death by arteriosclerosis could change under war conditions. Or, with effort, one can also imagine a genetic bias in a population so that people who migrate at any one time may be just those genetically predisposed to arteriosclerosis.

In the tradition of such skepticism, one could argue that while smokers suffer a higher incidence of hypertension, lung cancer, coronary disease, and emphysema than nonsmokers, this is not because of the effects of smoking but instead, because people with a predisposition to smoke are also the kind prone to lung cancer, coronary disease, and so on. This statement certainly appears to be a rationalization, but it is a logical possibility and is not easily refuted. In part, the limitations of epidemiological studies emerge from the inescapable necessity of acquiring data passively, without being able to perform controlled experiments such as depriving addicted smokers of cigarettes while keeping track of changes in their health.

In summary, arteriosclerosis is a disease of the blood vessels of people and animals. It has been with our species for thousands of years. Pathological studies in developed countries show that a majority of people, from infants to old people, have arteries with arteriosclerosis. There are exceptional groups, however, who show that it is possible to live with very little disease. In addition, genetically similar populations experience drastic shifts in incidence of atherosclerosis upon migration or during periods of national emergency. Such facts indicate that environmental factors cause the disease.

In our next chapter we chronicle a 70-year attempt on the part of many investigators to formulate an understanding of the features of arteriosclerosis. The work was done mainly in the laboratory, not in the field. The hypothesis spawned by these laboratory studies is recognizable as today's conservative explanation for the disease. As we will argue, it has failed to account for the origin and cause of arteriosclerosis, although it has had powerful influence on how the disease is diagnosed and treated.

CHAPTER 2
The Cholesterol Hypothesis

IT IS COMMON KNOWLEDGE that we eat too much animal fat, and everybody seems to know that this leads to arteriosclerosis. Television ads for corn oil extoll its lack of cholesterol. A U.S. Senate subcommittee on American nutrition recently recommended that Americans reduce dietary animal fat. There is a new method of French cooking called *nouvelle cuisine* built upon the principle of reducing fatty ingredients. A supermarket executive came out of retirement to rescue the school lunch program of Clark County, Nevada, with such innovations as hot dogs made of turkey meat and milk shakes made of algae. He received the Outstanding Achievement Award of the Nevada Heart Association, not because of his culinary creativity but because his nutritious lunches were low in cholesterol. A link between the intake of high cholesterol foods and heart disease is a concept that doctors and laymen share. But is it true?

Surprising as it may seem, cholesterol is no rare poison ingested only in fats such as butter. As every biochemist knows, cholesterol is universally present in sizable quantities as a structural component in the membranes of all animal cells. Cholesterol belongs to the broad category of *lipids*, molecules made up of chains of carbon and hydrogen atoms; lipids do not dissolve in water. Cholesterol travels through the watery environment of the blood by combining with protein to form *lipoproteins*, which are water-soluble.

All human cells can make cholesterol, although most is made by the liver. Diet accounts for a relatively small fraction of the total amount of cholesterol in the body. Cholesterol

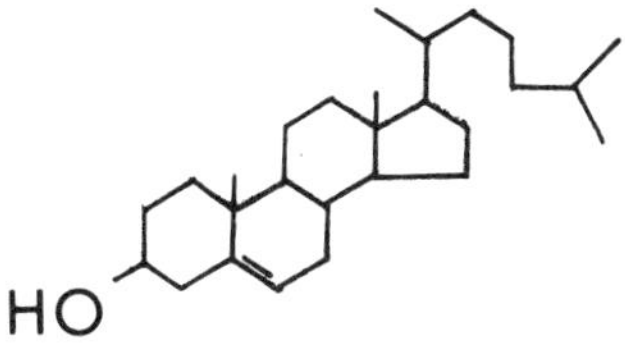

cholesterol

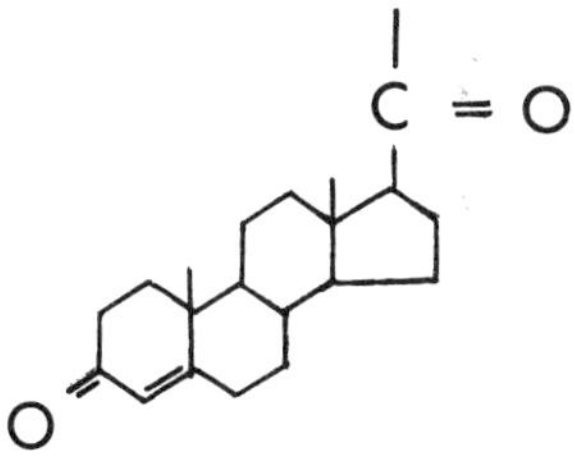

progesterone

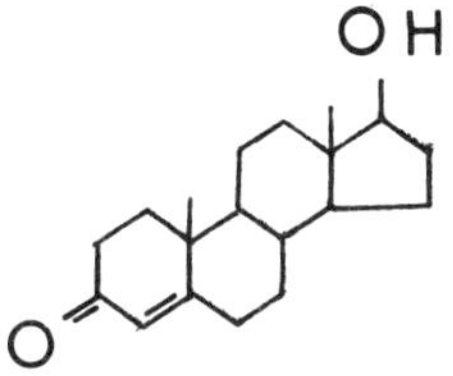

testosterone

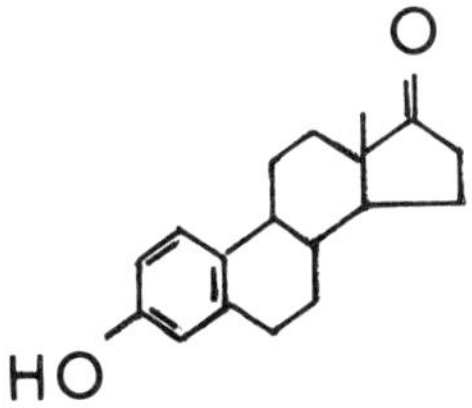

estrone
(an estrogen)

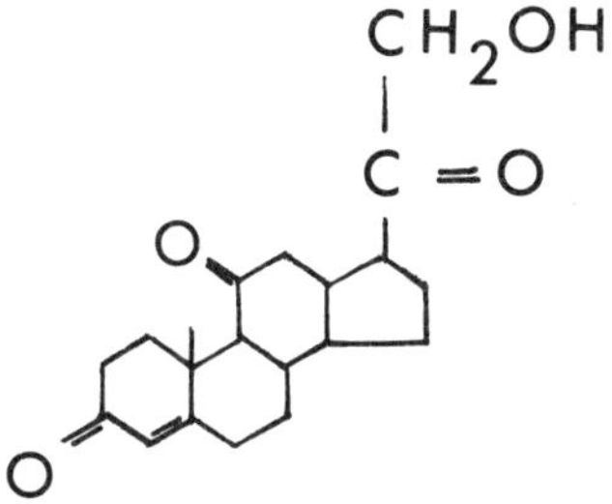

cortisone

Cholesterol shares a similar structure with other molecules produced by the body (after Mahler and Cordes 1971).

has the basic four-ringed configuration shared by steroid hormones such as estrogens, testosterone, and bile acids. The liver not only manufactures cholesterol, it also uses the compound to make bile acids for the digestive tract. Dietary intake influences the rate of the body's cholesterol production. If we eat less cholesterol, our bodies produce more. Even people who eat no cholesterol, such as vegetarians, produce significant amounts of cholesterol, which can then be found in their blood and body tissues.

DEVELOPMENT OF THE CHOLESTEROL HYPOTHESIS

How is it that this ubiquitous molecule has become so widely implicated as a cause of arteriosclerosis? We will trace our present notions from their origins in scientific investigations performed in Tsarist Russia at the turn of the century.

Working at the Imperial Academy of Medicine in St. Petersburg, A.I. Ignatovski studied records covering a 60-year period, showing that a rise in arteriosclerosis in England and France had paralleled the rise in per capita consumption of meat. He hypothesized that the protein in the meat caused the disease, an idea he tested by feeding rabbits various amounts of meat, eggs, and milk. Ignatovski first reported his results in 1908, showing that all rabbits fed animal protein developed arteriosclerotic aortas.

Ignatovski's work was of great importance because he was the first to demonstrate that merely changing diet could cause arteriosclerosis. The field of dietary induction of arteriosclerosis dates from his work.

Other Russian investigators accepted Ignatovski's results, but did not agree with his interpretation that the protein in the diet caused the disease. Surely, they argued, there are constituents besides protein in meat, eggs, and milk. Dr. Stuckey who, like Ignatovski, worked in St. Petersburg, found that rabbits fed egg yolk became arteriosclerotic. He concluded, therefore, that something in egg yolk caused the disease. Several subsequent discoveries lent support to this view. Chalatow, from the same

Institute as Ignatovski, discovered that by feeding egg yolk to rabbits, their liver cells accumulated fatty substances, particularly cholesterol. He and his colleague N. Anitschkow next fed rabbits a diet containing pure cholesterol dissolved in oil. Within a few weeks the rabbits' livers were infiltrated with cholesterol and they had atheromas within their aortas. Thus, cholesterol seemed to cause arteriosclerosis and this explained the previous results of Ignatovski and Stuckey: cholesterol was a common factor in all the diets that had caused lesions. From this point in 1913 until today, cholesterol has played the central role in dietary explanations of arteriosclerosis.

Anitschkow, who later became Professor of Histology at the University of Leningrad, went on to do much work on the subject of cholesterol-induced arteriosclerosis. In a review paper (1933) published 20 years after his initial discovery, he summed up his observations on the disease: "Atherosclerosis is not essentially of degenerative nature but rather of an infiltrative character. . . . The process always begins with the accumulation of lipoid substance of the innermost layers of the arterial wall. . . . Feeding with the cholesterin [cholesterol] is the only method which makes it possible for us to produce in certain species of animals changes that may be regarded as equivalent to those typical of human atherosclerosis."

EARLY PROBLEMS WITH THE CHOLESTEROL HYPOTHESIS

In 1913, the same year that Chalatow and Anitschkow published their influential results, two investigators from the University of Munich undertook an experiment in which they fed rabbits a mixture of oats and cholesterol. While some rabbits did develop arteriosclerosis, the investigators found no relationship between the amount of cholesterol in the diet and the severity of the ensuing arteriosclerosis. For instance, the rabbit that had eaten cholesterol for the longest time and that had the highest blood cholesterol level had a normal aorta.

These observations made it difficult to explain how cholesterol could be the direct cause of the disease. It was also known, even at the time of Chalatow and Anitschkow, that local injuries to blood vessels by artificial mechanical abrasion caused deposition of cholesterol within days or weeks. Thus mechanical damage alone could cause deposition of cholesterol in the arterial wall even when no cholesterol had been added to the diet.

In those cases in which cholesterol did appear to cause the disease, what could be the mechanism? The diets in these experiments were highly unusual for the animals. In 1915 a German scientist showed that if rabbits were fed a normal diet with large supplements of cholesterol, they did not develop arteriosclerosis. But rabbits fed abnormal diets with one-fifteenth the amount of cholesterol supplement did get arteriosclerosis. He concluded that cholesterol *per se* did not cause the disease. The disease, he reasoned, was the result of some other aspect of the abnormal diet.

Anitschkow and others who promulgated the cholesterol hypothesis read the results of the contradictory experiments. But the news did not seem to disturb them. After all, the central tenets had not been contradicted. The rule remained true that high cholesterol in the rabbit diet usually led to elevated cholesterol levels in the blood, and when the animal became arteriosclerotic, there was cholesterol in the lesion. Any other hypothesis than the one that dietary cholesterol caused the lesion seemed more complicated. The cholesterol people did not, however, perform direct experiments to rule out Ignatovski's original hypothesis that animal protein caused the disease.

DIETARY PROTEIN

Only a handful of subsequent investigators continued to take seriously the possible relationship between animal protein and arteriosclerosis. We will describe their work both because it will help us sharpen our assessment of the cholesterol hypothesis and because it lays the foundation for an alternative view of the cause of arteriosclerosis. The most prominent and persistent of the investigators were Dr. L. H. Newburgh and his colleagues (1923) at the University of Michigan Medical School who studied various effects of protein in the diet of rabbits. They fed two groups of rabbits high animal protein/low cholesterol diets; one diet contained 27 percent protein, the other diet contained 36 percent protein. They found that animal protein could indeed cause arteriosclerosis. Animals eating the 36 percent protein diet became arteriosclerotic earlier than the animals eating the 27 percent protein diet. Newburgh's group observed that the "occurrence and extent of atherosclerosis was roughly proportional" to the number of days the rabbits spent on the diet. Newburgh gave the experimental diets for shorter periods of time than those used for producing lesions by administering cholesterol. Furthermore, the cholesterol content in both of Newburgh's experimental diets was much lower than the cholesterol levels other investigators needed to produce arteriosclerosis. The brief exposures to dietary cholesterol and its low levels made it impossible to account for the arteriosclerosis solely on the basis of cholesterol.

With distinct open-mindedness, Newburgh's group did investigate the role of cholesterol (Clarkson and Newburgh 1926). They confirmed that diets high enough in cholesterol could cause arteriosclerosis, but in agreement with earlier investigators, they discovered no significant relation between level of blood cholesterol and amounts of cholesterol ingested. Newburgh's group also discovered that feeding rabbits a high protein/low cholesterol diet resulted in high cholesterol levels in the blood despite the low levels of cholesterol in the diet. Diets with lower protein and the same cholesterol level led to no such increase in serum cholesterol (when fed to control groups). The clear interpretation of the findings was that when the rabbits ate protein, they synthesized more of their own cholesterol. From this conclusion Newburgh posed the following puzzle: "The question immediately arises whether the atherosclerosis is caused by the hypercholesterolemia [high blood cholesterol] in this series of rabbits, or whether the two abnormalities occur concomitantly and do not bear the relation of cause and effect to each other, or finally whether the aortic disease occasions the [high blood cholesterol]."

Anitschkow (1933) defended the cholesterol hypothesis against Newburgh but made no test of dietary protein himself: "Some authors have even advanced the view that protein is a more important factor in the genesis of atherosclerosis than cholesterin [cholesterol], but this is undoubtedly an erroneous assumption, because very severe atherosclerotic changes can be produced by feeding with pure [cholesterol] without protein." Anitschkow did not dismiss animal protein entirely as a possible cause of arteriosclerosis, but he insisted on the primacy of cholesterol.

There was a logical standoff between those who believed in cholesterol and those who believed in animal protein as the cause of arteriosclerosis. There is no question that dietary cholesterol, in large enough quantities, under certain conditions, can cause arteriosclerosis. But the amounts required are indeed substantial. Dr. G.C. Frank and colleagues at Louisiana State University Medical School (1978) have pointed out that the concentration of cholesterol needed to induce arteriosclerosis is at least ten times the concentration found in human diets. In a well-known study, for example, Dr. Dragoslava Vesselinovitch and colleagues at the University of Chicago (1976) induced arteriosclerosis in monkeys with a cholesterol diet. The diet, however, contained extraordinarily high levels of cholesterol (2 percent plus 25 percent fat) for 18 months. The maximum level of cholesterol in normal human diets is around 0.2 percent.

Another problem with the cholesterol hypothesis is that in humans, dietary cholesterol is not easily absorbed through the intestine. In fact, as mentioned earlier, biochemists have shown that most of the cholesterol found in body tissue is synthesized by the body out of smaller molecules. When dietary intake is low, the body synthesizes more cholesterol; when intake is high the rate of synthesis declines.

Despite such problems, the cholesterol notion has predominated so completely that today protein enjoys the highest dietary respectability. The possibility that protein is a culprit in arteriosclerosis has dropped out of our daily consciousness. Possibly the weak spots in the cholesterol hypothesis went unemphasized because of enthusiasm for the neatness of both the explanation for the disease and the prescribed treatment in the form of low-cholesterol diets. It seemed clear that high diet cholesterol led to increased serum cholesterol which in turn led to the formation of atheromas. Furthermore, no one could explain clearly the mechanism by which protein could act to produce arteriosclerosis. Whatever the reason, neither argument held sufficient scientific strength to resolve the debate. But an accident of scientific history tipped the balance against advocates of the protein hypothesis.

DISASTER FOR THE PROTEIN HYPOTHESIS

What substance could be in animal protein that could cause arteriosclerosis? That was the question Newburgh posed in 1924. Proteins are collections of *amino acids* that are strung together linearly like beads. Newburgh assumed that one or more of the amino acids must be toxic and produce atheromas. In a series of experiments, he showed that some amino acids were mildly toxic, others not at all. But no amino acid was dramatically toxic (Newburgh and Marsh 1925). The matter rested there.

The investigators had stalled on the verge of a dramatic finding, which had eluded them because of unlucky historical timing. They had tested all 15 of the amino acids available in 1924, the last of which had been discovered in 1904. Biochemists doing protein research suspected that other amino acids existed, but the chemical techniques used at that time to isolate amino acids involved a step that prevented the purification and identification of certain sulfur-containing amino acids. New developments in biochemistry were required and it wasn't until 1922 that J.H. Mueller discovered *methionine*. This new sulfur-containing amino acid was not available as a pure substance until after Newburgh's group had completed its investigations. Thus, methionine was not tested in the 1920s.

The failure to find a critical amino acid was a historical near-miss, one that permitted the consolidation of the cholesterol hypothesis. Later work, discussed in Chapter 4, has shown that homocysteine, a by-product of methionine metabolism, rapidly causes extensive and severe arteriosclerosis. Newburgh's methods would have been adequate to discover that methionine in dietary protein produces the disease. But Newburgh abandoned the search for toxic amino acids in 1926, although he maintained an interest in the problem of arteriosclerosis and was a strong critic of the cholesterol hypothesis for many years.

After 1930 the animal protein hypothesis of arteriosclerosis nearly dropped out of scientific consideration as investigators concentrated their attention on cholesterol. However, occasional reports showed that interest was still alive. In 1941 Dr. Dorothy Meeker and Dr. Homer Kesten of the Department of Pathology of Columbia University Medical School read the Newburgh group's studies and were concerned that since a small amount of cholesterol had been mixed with the animal protein fed to the rabbits, perhaps the cholesterol had caused the arteriosclerosis. Meeker and Kesten repeated the Newburgh experiments, but took precautions to eliminate *all* cholesterol in the protein they fed to their rabbits. Their results nonetheless confirmed Newburgh: even with no cholesterol in the diet, they found high levels of blood cholesterol and arteriosclerotic aortas having lesions that were "indistinguishable from those produced by cholesterol." They also observed that other rabbits fed an equivalent amount of vegetable protein in the form of soy flour developed no arteriosclerosis. This intriguing finding indicates that protein-containing foods differ in toxicity. Later work has revealed the basis of this difference, and we discuss it in Chapter 7. The importance of Meeker and Kesten's work is that it shows animal protein alone, with no cholesterol, is a sufficient cause of arteriosclerosis.

But such experiments were rare. With the apparent dead-end hit by Newburgh's group, who were unable to find a strongly toxic amino acid, cholesterol remained the plausible dietary candidate. It had not been conclusively proven, but it appealed strongly to clinicians and others who needed a working explanation. Animal protein slowly slipped out of the picture. In 1933 Anitschkow, the cholesterol advocate, felt compelled to mention Newburgh's protein work before dismissing it. However, in a review paper prepared for publication in 1967, Anitschkow no longer cited Newburgh's work. Like certain items in previous editions of Russian encyclopedias but currently out of favor, Newburgh's work quite simply disappeared. In the same period, the cholesterol hypothesis began to garner confirmatory epidemiological evidence.

Implicit in the thinking of both camps was the idea that, as with tuberculosis, or malaria, or any well understood disease, arteriosclerosis had a single cause. After the work of Anitschkow and the others, the vast majority of investigators believed that dietary cholesterol was that sole cause.

EPIDEMIOLOGY OF CHOLESTEROL AND THE CASE FOR THE CHOLESTEROL HYPOTHESIS

During those 30 years, with the single exception of Eskimos, peoples who had high-cholesterol intake were found to suffer higher rates of coronary heart disease than populations which had low-cholesterol intake. We have noted how well the Bedouins fit this concept, since their dietary cholesterol is extremely low and their rate of heart disease is practically zero. The Tukisenta in New Guinea consume virtually no cholesterol. They have very low serum cholesterol levels and have only a slight incidence of coronary heart disease. Furthermore, vegetarians have low-cholesterol intake, low serum levels, and low risk of heart attack. And epidemiologists, having noted that Japanese moving from Japan to Hawaii to California developed a progressive tendency toward coronary heart disease, also learned that the level of serum cholesterol underwent a parallel increase.

In addition, the risk of coronary heart disease was shown to correlate strongly with the level of serum cholesterol. The results confirm a strong association between cholesterol in the serum and risk of arteriosclerotic disease. Recent medical practice has drawn from this association the therapeutic recommendation that individuals should reduce their consumption of dietary cholesterol. It is argued that such reduction will result in lower levels of cholesterol in the serum. In turn, the reduction in serum cholesterol is expected to lessen the risk of arteriosclerotic disease.

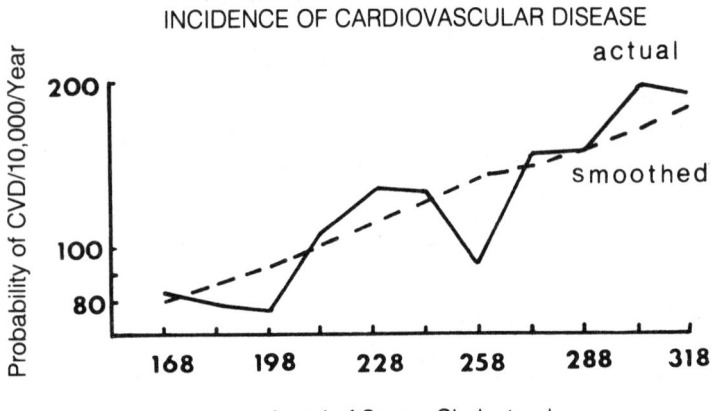

This graph shows how the yearly incidence of cardiovascular disease (per 10,000 people) rises with serum cholesterol level: based on men and women aged 45 to 64 years (from Kannel et al., 1976).

The appeal of this argument is strong. The following chart is based on clinical statistics giving the risks associated with high-serum cholesterol as well as other factors. For a patient having none of the risk factors listed, the probability of developing coronary heart disease in an eight-year period is well below average. High serum cholesterol triples his risk. Other factors, such as diabetes, smoking, and an enlarged heart, add still more to the risk. (Women show a similar trend, but have less than half the risk of men in most categories.)

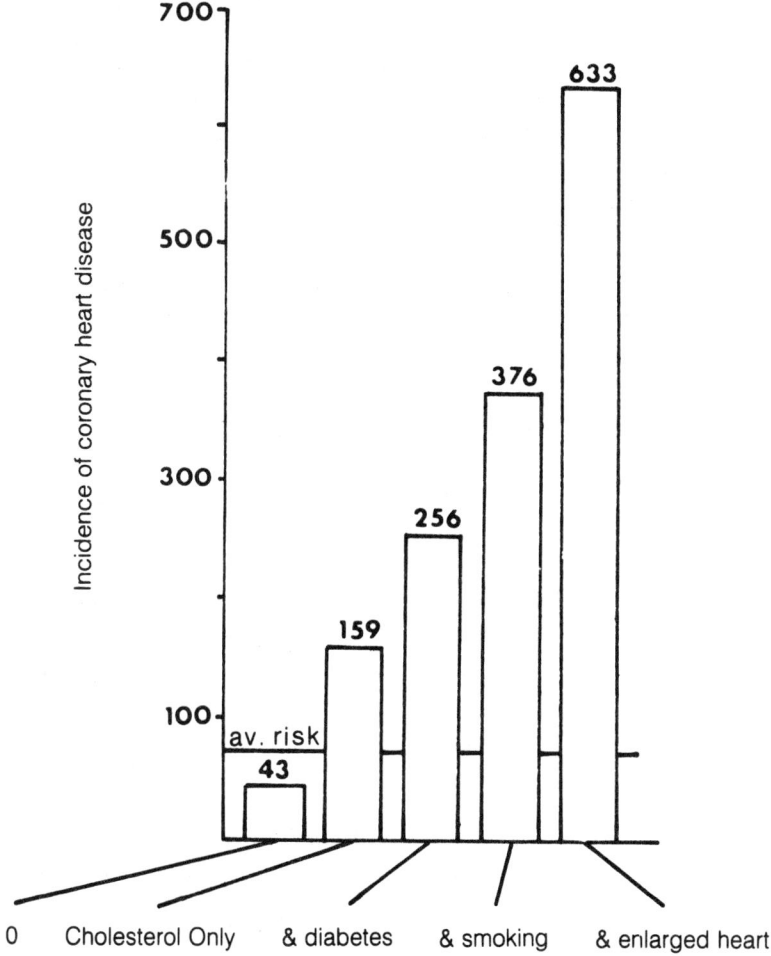

The chart shows how incidence of coronary heart disease rises in men having increasing numbers of risk factors. (Number of cases in a span of eight years per 1,000 men all with normal blood pressure—below 150 mm Hg) (from Kannel et al. 1976).

By the 1950s, emphasis had shifted from cholesterol as *the* cause to cholesterol as the most important of several risk factors. Today management of arteriosclerosis is guided more by the notion of minimizing risks. By looking at arteriosclerosis from the point of view of risk factors, researchers can tolerate ambiguities about the effects of cholesterol. In practice, the cloud of risk factors obscures the significance of cases in which low-cholesterol, low-fat dietary therapy has been ineffective. Recently, there has been a 20 percent decrease in coronary mortality. But there is virtually no evidence to show that low cholesterol diets were responsible, despite claims to that effect.

There has been rather vigorous questioning and defending of the scientific basis of dietary therapy. Dr. George Mann's controversial article, quoted in our introduction, elicited so much correspondence that the editors of the *New England Journal of Medicine* allowed the Nutrition Committee of the American Heart Association to present its case for cholesterol diet therapy. The resulting article (Glueck et al. 1978), which the editors considered "balanced and well-documented," reviewed both established and recent evidence. It singled out a 1964 study that appeared in the *Journal of Clinical Investigation* to buttress the authors' contention that "six decades of evidence have provided a considerable degree of certainty that the level of plasma cholesterol is determined by the intake of dietary cholesterol, saturated and polyunsaturated fat, and total calories."

The study they quote (Connor et al. 1964), however, lasted four months and was based on only six men of average weight, three of whom were diabetics and one of whom did not complete the study. Over the course of the study, the group followed four different diets, each for a month, switching after each month to the next diet. Two diets contained no cholesterol and two were high in cholesterol, with varied amounts of *polyunsaturated* and *saturated fat*.

After one month on high-cholesterol intake, the subjects were switched to a zero-cholesterol diet having roughly the same fat composition. The average level of serum cholesterol dropped from 213 to 175 mg (or almost 18 percent). The subjects maintained the zero-cholesterol intake, while fats were lowered during the third dietary period, but this made no difference in average serum cholesterol of the five remaining subjects. However, cholesterol intake was raised again during the fourth month's diet while the saturated fats were held low; the average serum cholesterol of the fourth-period blood samples rose to 202 (16 percent).

The authors of this study concluded that dietary cholesterol "influenced greatly the serum cholesterol . . . levels in six men." They also cited studies of other small groups, but none of these showed any stronger relation between diet and serum cholesterol, nor did they show the clinical worth of dietary therapy.

HDL AND LDL

The nutrition committee also discussed a recent refinement of the cholesterol story. Since cholesterol is not soluble in the blood, it must be carried by attachment to soluble *lipoprotein* molecules. Cholesterol can be bound to the lipoproteins of high density*(HDL)* and to those of low density *(LDL)*. Populations that are low in risk of coronary heart disease have HDL-cholesterol in higher concentration. Some physicians therefore ascribe a protective effect to cholesterol bound to HDL. Conversely, cholesterol bound to LDL is correlated with high risk of arteriosclerosis. (It has also been found that on the average, the higher HDL-cholesterol is, the lower LDL-cholesterol is; the two types antagonize each other.) So instead of lowering all serum cholesterol, a new therapeutic approach is to lower LDL-cholesterol while boosting HDL-cholesterol. Much present research consists of studies indicating how this new goal might be accomplished by reducing smoking, by exercising, and by reducing the level of cholesterol or carbohydrates in the diet.

The "protection effect" of HDL-cholesterol in coronary heart disease is shown in the following graph drawn from pooled results of the five largest studies of heart disease in the United

States, carried out on more than 6,000 people over a period of many years (Castelli et al. 1977). The graph applies for all patients between the ages of 50 and 69. The data shows a weak but statistically significant inverse relation between HDL-cholesterol level and presence of coronary heart disease: higher HDL-cholesterol, lower rate of coronary heart disease.

This modification of the cholesterol hypothesis does not point toward a cure. Dr. George Mann has shown that measuring serum HDL- and LDL-cholesterol instead of measuring total serum cholesterol has failed even to improve detection of people at high risk. The Nutrition Committee of the American Heart Association offered only the hope that lowering cholesterol in children might be more effective than it has been in adults. They observed that the recent 20 percent drop in coronary heart disease parallels a diminishing intake of cholesterol since 1970. Nonetheless, they admit that correlation is

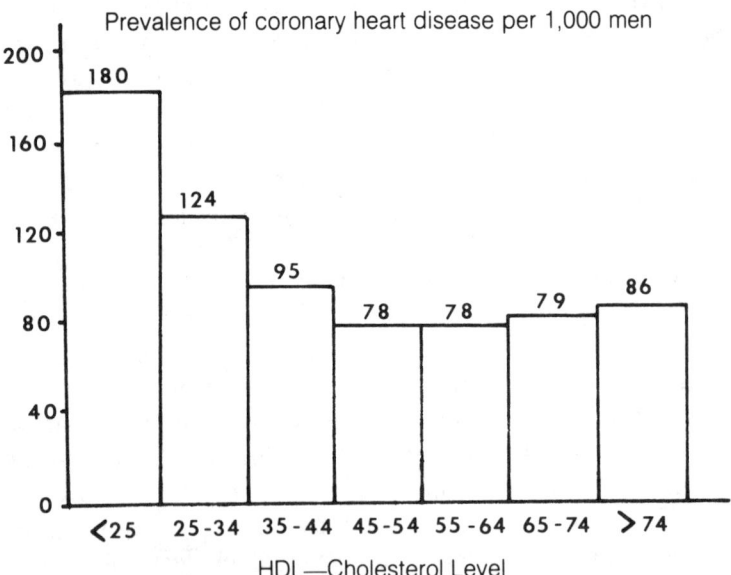

This chart shows the relation between the prevalence of coronary heart disease and HDL-cholesterol level in men aged 50 to 69 (from Castelli et al., 1978).

not cause, and that recent shifts in cholesterol intake are accompanied by other changes in diet. In the end, their rebuttal to Mann was equivocal. They stressed that dietary therapy is in itself safe, and hoped that ongoing studies of risk factors will eventually lead to a resolution of the question of whether or not dietary therapy is effective. The equivocal conclusion after 60 years of work is an indication of the need for a new way to look at the data.

CHOLESTEROL AND ANIMAL PROTEIN

Before we look closely at tests of the cholesterol hypothesis, we want to point out that data from surveys linking dietary cholesterol and heart disease also link diets high in animal protein with heart disease. Though much is made of the Bedouins' low dietary cholesterol, for example, they also have quite low intakes of animal protein. There is, of course, a close link between dietary cholesterol and dietary animal protein (foods, such as milk and beef, that have one also have the other). It is quite intriguing to observe how some epidemiologists, aware of this link, have carefully avoided the appearance of endorsing the fallen notion that animal protein is a possible cause of disease. For instance, J. Yerushalmy and H. Hilleboe of the School of Public Health, University of California, Berkeley, and the New York State Department of Health, Albany, wrote in 1957: "It must be emphatically stated that the authors do not intend to suggest that the association between dietary protein and heart disease is valid . . . the data are presented to illustrate the steps necessary to test the 'specificity' of the dietary fat–heart disease association." But these authors also went on to say, "The data . . . do not support the view that dietary fat is uniquely or unequivocally associated with mortality from heart disease."

In 1959 N. Jolliffe and M. Archer of the Bureau of Nutrition of the New York City Department of Health made a statistical study of arteriosclerosis and observed a high correlation between the disease and saturated fats. There was also a high correlation with animal protein. "This may be explained," they wrote, "by the fact that land mammal meats are carriers of fat, by the close affinity between intakes of milk proteins and butterfat and by the effects of close association between intakes of fish proteins and marine oils. . . ."

Nevin Scrimshaw and M. Guzman of the Massachusetts Institute of Technology and Instituto de Nutricion de Centro America y Panama wrote in 1968: "A strong positive correlation of animal protein consumption was observed [in our study] because this dietary variable closely paralleled the fat calories; it was not considered etiologically important because of the supporting evidence for a primary role of fat, rather than protein, in determining levels of serum cholesterol, severity of atherosclerosis, and incidence of coronary heart disease."

These examples indicate that there is a climate of endorsement of the cholesterol hypothesis sufficiently strong that it influences the presentation of research results. There are no signs that the above authors felt compelled to undertake the investigations necessary to probe the significance of their own findings concerning animal protein even though such experiments could be done unambiguously. Does modern evidence justify the tendency to accept the cholesterol hypothesis?

CLINICAL TESTS OF CHOLESTEROL

The cholesterol hypothesis consists of a logical chain of three major testable predictions. First, diet, particularly foods high in cholesterol, should affect the level of cholesterol in blood serum. Second, reducing serum cholesterol should reduce coronary mortality. Third, the severity of arteriosclerosis should be related to the level of serum cholesterol.

DIET AND SERUM CHOLESTEROL

The relation of diet to serum cholesterol has been investigated in the Framingham Study, one of the most extensive (and famous) long-term studies of cardiovascular disease. The principal aim of the Framingham Study is to determine the extent to which heart disease develops in individual subjects over a period of many years. Six thousand people, all between ages 30 and 59, were originally chosen from the town of Framingham, Massachusetts. Begun in 1948, the study continues today under the aegis of the National Institutes of Health; there have been more than 30 substudies devoted to different questions concerned with heart disease.

One aspect of this enormous study was to determine the effect of diet on serum cholesterol. A subgroup of 900 individuals were checked every three months, for a period of four years, to find out what they were eating (Kannel and Gordon 1970). (Investigators recorded the intake of animal fat, vegetable fat, protein, cholesterol, *complex* and *simple carbohydrates*, and total calories.) Blood samples were taken and the level of serum cholesterol measured for each person. The result was quite simple: The first prediction of the cholesterol hypothesis was not supported. The investigators concluded: "There is a considerable range of serum cholesterol levels within the Framingham Study Group. Something explains this inter-individual variation, but it is not diet (as measured here)."

The investigation found that serum cholesterol was *not* related to cholesterol intake in food or to fat consumption.

The Framingham study, although the most famous, is consistent with other investigations that have also found little relation between diet cholesterol and serum cholesterol. A group at the University of Michigan Schools of Medicine and Public Health studied the diets of 4,000 men and women in Tecumseh, Michigan, and found a similar lack of association between dietary fat and serum cholesterol levels (Nichols et al. 1976). In Jerusalem, among 10,000 male civil service employees, there was also very low correlation between dietary elements, "which included total fat, saturated fat, various fatty acids and serum cholesterol" (Kahn et al. 1969).

A group headed by G. C. Frank (1978) at the Department of Medicine at Louisiana State University Medical Center in New Orleans wondered if previous studies of adults had failed to detect the correlation between serum and dietary levels of cholesterol because adults were too far along in the disease to show profound differences. So they chose to study children instead. They examined the diets of 194 ten-year-olds in Bogalusa, Louisiana, and additionally measured not only serum levels of total cholesterol, but the cholesterol carried by both high- and low-density lipoproteins. The investigators found that no dietary component in these children's diets "accounted for more than 4 percent of the variability in the risk factor parameter, leaving 96 percent of the variability unexplained."

And in a smaller study in Evans County, Georgia, using 26 matched pairs of people with high- and low-serum cholesterol, researchers found that dietary variables (including fat, saturated fat, and fatty acids) did not correlate significantly with serum cholesterol values (Stulb et al. 1965).

All of these studies belie the commonly held belief that high diet cholesterol leads to high serum cholesterol. The studies mentioned earlier that showed a relationship between diet cholesterol and serum cholesterol were much smaller and less conclusive than these that failed to corroborate such a relation. As we noted, even the most favorable findings show less than 20 percent changes in serum cholesterol level as a result of a controlled diet.

Of course, even if diet did strictly control serum cholesterol, dietary therapy might still be ineffective against arteriosclerosis. There is an obvious appeal to reduce risk factors once their tight correlation to a disease is seen, but there is no *logical* reason to expect the technique to work. Measles spots are obviously correlated with measles and fever is associated with pneumonia. But nobody would expect that elimination of the spots (say, by surgery) would cure measles, or that cooling of the body would cure pneumonia. Reduction of serum cholesterol would be expected to work only if cholesterol really *caused* human arteriosclerosis.

Additional experimental work has confirmed the major epidemiological studies' finding that dietary changes do *not* produce significant changes of cholesterol level in the blood.

What if cholesterol were added to the diet? Margaret Flynn and colleagues, affiliated with several medical schools, studied this question by exploring the effect of adding cholesterol to a diet of healthy American adults (Porter et al. 1977). They allowed 114 male volunteers (average age 45 years) to eat their customary diets but restricted certain high-cholesterol foods. The average daily content of cholesterol in their diets was 301 mg. For 12 weeks 55 of these volunteers (Group 1) ate an additional whole egg daily, giving them a total daily intake of cholesterol of 536 mg. The other 59 subjects ate no whole egg for the same period (Group II). Then, for the second 12-week period, Group I ate no whole eggs and each member of Group II ate a whole egg daily. The conclusion of the study was that there was "no significant influence of dietary regimen on serum cholesterol," despite a whopping 78 percent increase in dietary cholesterol. The study was repeated two years later. This time the high diet cholesterol group ate two whole eggs daily (Flynn et al. 1979). The results were still the same: "We found no significant increase in serum cholesterol with dietary intake of two eggs daily for 3 months. . . ."

An even more severe test was made in New Guinea, where Dr. Malcolm Whyte and fellow researchers from Australian National University and the Papua New Guinea Institute of Medical Research studied the Tukisenta, who live in the area of Goroka in the central highlands of Papua, New Guinea. The Tukisenta, as noted in Chapter 1, have a very low rate of cardiovascular disease. In addition, their diet is "practically free of fat and cholesterol. . . ." For five weeks Whyte supplemented the normal diet of the Tukisenta with a daily ration of omelettes made from reconstituted egg yolks containing 1,000 mg (!) cholesterol. Before, during, and after the high-cholesterol period, Whyte measured serum cholesterol. His group found that "plasma cholesterol levels showed no significant differences between the two control and the cholesterol periods." Thus, epidemiological studies and clinical tests invalidate the notion that high diet cholesterol leads to high serum cholesterol.

LEVEL OF SERUM CHOLESTEROL VERSUS CORONARY MORTALITY

The second prediction of the cholesterol hypothesis is that if serum cholesterol could be reduced, coronary mortality should decrease. In a major investigation, the Coronary Drug Project, which was conducted in 1975 in 52 clinics across the country, two groups of 1,000 male coronary patients were given drugs that reduce serum cholesterol. (The drugs, clofibrate and niacin, reduced serum cholesterol by 6.5 percent and 9.9 percent, respectively.) Even with this reduction, which was statistically significant, there was no statistically significant difference in coronary mortality between patients on these drugs and 3,000 other coronary patients who received *placebos*. Thus, changing cholesterol level did not affect mortality in this study, nor has it been shown to do so in other recent work.

RELATION BETWEEN SERUM CHOLESTEROL AND SEVERITY OF ATHEROSCLEROSIS

Third, the cholesterol hypothesis suggests that the severity of arteriosclerosis should be related to the level of serum cholesterol. The higher the level, the more severe the arteriosclerosis. The best way to determine the extent of obstruction of coronary blood vessels is to remove them, section them into very thin slices, and examine them under a microscope. (Obviously, this procedure is restricted to arteries from dead people.) While people are alive, there is an alternative method for measuring the arterial lumen without removing the artery. An opaque substance is added to the blood of the coronary arteries and the heart is X-rayed. At each place where an atheroma restricts flow of blood, the opaque stream will narrow. If the vessel is blocked, no opacity will show up downstream.

The procedure, called arteriography, is highly revealing but it is a surgical operation and carries some risks. Because of this, it is not done routinely, but only on people showing clinical signs of coronary disease. As a test of the severity of arteriosclerosis, arteriography is excellent.

At the Mayo Clinic, arteriographies were given to 300 patients with symptoms of serious coronary heart disease. During their stay at the clinic these patients' serum lipids, including cholesterol, were also measured (Fuster et al. 1975). It was found that "when patients with [high lipid levels] were compared with patients with normal serum lipid concentrations, the number, distribution, and degree of vessels diseased were found to be similar. . . . The presence or absence of . . . [high lipid levels] . . . was not correlated with the coronary anatomical patterns."

In other words, high serum cholesterol was not associated with more severe arteriosclerosis than low serum cholesterol. The cholesterol hypothesis thus failed to meet another critical test.

The tests we have described do not contradict the fact that people with high serum cholesterol have a high risk of coronary heart disease. The correlation between cholesterol and heart disease has been found in many studies, including the Framingham Study. It is now known, for example, that a man 30 to 39 years old with serum cholesterol above 259 mg per 100 cc is 300 percent more prone to coronary heart disease than a similar man whose cholesterol level is below 200.

Yet such dramatic correlation does not prove that cholesterol causes arteriosclerosis any more than spots cause measles. Instead, these investigations—the epidemiological studies, the cholesterol diet studies, the Coronary Drug Project, and the Mayo Clinic Arteriography Study—provide important evidence against predictions of the cholesterol hypothesis.

We have seen that the level of diet cholesterol has little relation to the level of serum cholesterol; reducing serum cholesterol does not reduce coronary mortality; and the level of serum cholesterol is not related to severity of arteriosclerosis. These are not minor studies selected for rhetorical impact. They are major, extensive investigations which were intended to serve as a basis for medical practice.

It is still relevant to recall the questions Newburgh and his colleagues posed over fifty years ago: Is arteriosclerosis caused by the high serum cholesterol or do the two abnormalities occur concomitantly, without bearing any relation of cause and effect? Or does the aortic disease occasion the high serum cholesterol?

As early as 1935 Dr. G. Duff, a professor of pathology at the Johns Hopkins Medical School, after reviewing the preceding 25 years of research, concluded that high blood cholesterol did not cause arteriosclerosis. First, anticipating a far more contemporary point of view, he did not believe that the initial stage of the disease was the infiltration of cholesterol: "There is every reason to believe," he wrote, "that local injury to the walls [of the arteries] is an essential factor and the primary event in the development of arteriosclerosis in man." Second, he wrote, high serum cholesterol "is not found with any regularity in association with arteriosclerosis in man. . . . The only reason for suspecting [high serum cholesterol] as a factor in the etiology of human arteriosclerosis lies in the results of the cholesterol feeding experiments in rabbits. . . . In view of the data derived from the study of human material, it seems highly probable that arteriosclerosis in man can and usually does develop without deviation of the cholesterol content of the blood beyond the normal limits of variation."

In Duff's opinion, "All evidence which has been brought forward in the attempt to demonstrate a relationship between the cholesterol content of the diet and the development of arteriosclerosis in man is equivocal and therefore far from convincing. Indeed, it would hardly influence an opinion not already prejudiced in favor of the idea."

Then, writing in 1955, Dr. Meyer Friedman and colleagues reviewed several studies which showed that when coronary arteries are diseased but not yet occluded, there is a proliferation of cells and connective tissue in the intima, but cholesterol can not yet be detected in the lesion. Only at a later point can cholesterol be seen in the lesions.

Thus, it seems reasonable to answer Newburgh by saying that hypercholesterolemia does not lead to arteriosclerosis. People with high levels of serum cholesterol may indeed be found to be more likely to have arteriosclerosis. But this is not because serum cholesterol causes the disease; instead, high levels are simply associated in some way with the disease.

"Truth," said Leonardo da Vinci, "is the daughter of time, not authority." The cholesterol hypothesis has been around for over 60 years and has seemingly stood the test of time. But it is clear that the idea is a survivor, rather than a winner. It has accumulated a number of critics and defenders who are currently engaged in commenting on the hypothesis and who are attempting to influence the stalemated medical practices in this area.

DOUBTERS OF CHOLESTEROL HYPOTHESIS

In May 1980 a committee composed of 15 scientists and physicians of the Food and Nutrition Board of the National Research Council, issued a report, "Toward Healthful Diets" challenging the wisdom of lowering cholesterol in American diets.

> Although high serum cholesterol and LDL levels are positive risk factors for coronary disease, it has not been proven that lowering these levels by dietary intervention will consistently affect the rate of new coronary events. . . . No significant correlation between cholesterol intake and serum cholesterol concentration has been shown in free-living persons in this country. . . . For these reasons, the Board makes no specific recommendations about dietary cholesterol for the healthy person.

The report was front page news because the Food and Nutrition Board is a generally conservative group that sets recommended dietary allowances (RDAs) and comes under the auspices of the National Academy of Sciences.

Almost immediately there was strong negative reaction to the report. While no one contradicted the conclusions, the report was attacked because (a) it contained no new results, and (b) two of its members had received research and consulting money from industry egg boards. The presumption was that such people could not be objective. The Board members became the issue rather than the report itself.

The critics of the report appeared to apply a double standard to statements in support of and against low cholesterol diets. Dr. Robert Levy, the Director of the National Heart, Lung and

Blood Institute of the National Institutes of Health (N.I.H.), believes that a diet lower in cholesterol is a "prudent diet." Yet an investigator receiving money from the N.I.H. is not presumed biased because of Levy's opinions. At the same time, any scientific committee receiving some money from the egg industry is presumed biased.

Nicholas Wade (1980) of *Science* magazine commenting on the reaction to the report:

> The Academy has dared to utter an unpalatable truth, and has reaped the customary reward of those who challenge prevailing wisdom: abuse and obloquy, ad hominem attacks, ignorant sermons from the press, the yapping of offended special interests and the cant of discountenanced politicians. . . . The problem with the report lies not in its content—which has yet to be proved in error—but in its wrapping.

One critic of the cholesterol hypothesis, who does not accept any alternative hypothesis, is Dr. John McMichael of London. In 1976 the British Department of Health had circulated an advisory to all British doctors. The main recommendation was to lower plasma cholesterol by reducing saturated animal and dairy fat in the diet. McMichael, finding this recommendation "astonishing," wrote to the *Lancet,* a well-known British medical journal: "There can be little benefit on coronary incidence from such measures." He cited some of the evidence mentioned in this chapter and suggested that "we all have a degree of coronary atheroma after about age 30. It is only accidental complications that matter."

We part company with Dr. McMichael on this last point. What seems accidental and complex from the vantage point of the cholesterol hypothesis becomes far more interpretable when seen from a different point of view. In the following two chapters, we turn attention to the homocysteine theory and show how it accounts for the observations made by past researchers and provides an explanation of the disease.

CHAPTER 3

Vitamin B$_6$ Deficiency and Arteriosclerosis

B$_{\text{ECAUSE THE CHOLESTEROL HYPOTHESIS}}$ has not provided a satisfactory explanation of arteriosclerosis, early rejection of the protein hypothesis may have been premature. In this chapter, we turn to an entirely independent line of evidence distinguished from earlier concerns with either protein or cholesterol. The experiments are in the field of vitamins and nutrition. Although this appears to be a side issue, we will show that it is critically relevant to work relating protein to arteriosclerosis.

VITAMINS

The idea of vitamins, organic compounds needed in small amounts for good health, was first proposed in 1912. It was theorized that then common diseases, such as beriberi, scurvy, and rickets, were the results of specific chemical deficiencies, although at that time the physical structure of none of the hypothesized vitamins was known. Later, when specific vitamins were discovered, they were given letter designations. In some cases, when further research disclosed that what had originally seemed to be a single substance contained several independently active compounds, numbers were subscripted. By the 1920s, at about the time of Newburgh's studies, vitamin research had expanded into an important field.

THE DISCOVERY OF VITAMIN B$_6$

The first vitamin discovered was vitamin A, capping a search lasting centuries. In antiquity Egyptian and Greek physicians, including Hippocrates, had noted that eating liver could prevent "night blindness," an inability to see in dim light. From the perspective of the vitamin theory, their observation suggested that liver contained a specific compound that was in short supply in most other foods. Chemists isolated the compound in liver and designated it vitamin A. In 1929 they determined the structure of vitamin A. It was also learned that several foods contained vitamin A, needed to manufacture the light sensitive chemical necessary to see in dim light.

Scientists had also long suspected a nutritional cause for beriberi. Biochemists isolated a vitamin in 1926 that prevented beriberi and designated it vitamin B. A few years later, the structure of the compound was determined and vitamin B_1 was identified as thiamin. The subscript had to be added because other vitamins had since been found as a result of new extraction procedures. Nicotinic acid or niacin, which prevented pellagra, or black tongue, was named vitamin B_2.

Limes and other citrus fruits had been a compulsory ration for British sailors since 1804, but their scurvy-preventing compound was not isolated for more than a hundred years. In 1932 Dr. Albert Szent-Gyorgi extracted vitamin C from cabbages, oranges, and adrenal glands and confirmed that it was indeed the key to the antiscurvy (ascorbic) effect.

In 1934, two years after the isolation of vitamin C, Dr. Paul Gyorgy discovered the sixth separate B vitamin. Although vitamin B_6 (pyridoxine) is one of the cornerstones of the homocysteine theory of arteriosclerosis, it was initially distinguished from other B vitamins because it was the only factor that specifically prevented a peculiar form of dermatitis in rats.

By the end of the 1930s researchers had found that a variety of pathological conditions were caused by vitamin deficiencies. The initial discoveries linked individual vitamins to single illnesses such as vitamin C to scurvy, but with expanded research prompted by the dramatic cures, it became evident that most vitamins served multiple functions. Inadequate intake of single vitamins could lead to multiple pathologies affecting different organs or systems independently.

EXPERIMENTAL VITAMIN DEFICIENCY

In the 1940s Dr. James Rinehart and Dr. Louis Greenberg, two pathologists at the University of California Medical School in San Francisco, set out to examine the multiple metabolic and structural defects resulting from single vitamin deficiencies. Their subject was the rhesus monkey, a close relative to the human. It is similar in structure, biochemistry, and in its immune system.

Rinehart and Greenberg began their vitamin work with two studies: one on thiamin (vitamin B_1) deficiency and one on folic acid deficiency. The pathological results in both these studies were clear and they agreed with earlier clinical work. They led to no sweeping surprises, but they indicate that Rinehart and Greenberg were performing reliable experimental work.

VITAMIN B_6 DEFICIENCY AND VASCULAR LESIONS

Rinehart and Greenberg next turned their attention to a systematic study of vitamin B_6 deficiency. In this case the clinical manifestations were few and obscure. Dermatitis was the most commonly recognized consequence of vitamin B_6 deficiency, but there was no way to predict what additional pathologies might be found.

Early in their study the team realized they had made an important discovery. In pyridoxine deficiency "the most constant and prominent abnormality encountered" was "arterial lesions." They had maintained the animals with a diet deficient in vitamin B_6 for periods ranging from 5½ to 16 months. Even at 5½ months the researchers noted definite arterial changes. In animals kept 13 and 16 months they found prominent coronary artery lesions. "Small plaques of fibrous tissue developed in the intima . . . which bore a close resemblance to human lesions of arteriosclerosis . . . occurrence of the lesions at points [where arteries branch] was another feature of the experimental lesion common to the human disease."

Rinehart and Greenberg published several photographs of their results, including a color plate showing the fibrous thickenings and other pathologies they had observed. They were sure these results were breaking new ground and were obviously excited by the implications of their studies on how vitamin B$_6$-deficient diets could cause arteriosclerosis:

> There seems no question that the arterial lesions are related to pyridoxine deficiency. Such lesions have not developed in monkeys on the same dietary regime subjected to other dietary deficiencies and showing equal degrees of inanition [exhaustion of the body from not eating]. The experimental lesions which have been described have a close resemblance to arteriosclerosis as it occurs in man . . . it is noteworthy that prolonged feeding of cholesterol has failed to produce significant lesions in the monkey. This is in fact a potent argument against the cholesterol theory as a major influence in the pathogenesis of arteriosclerosis in man. As far as we know, the lesions here reported are the first of this type that have been described as resulting from deficiency of a specific food factor. The observation gains added significance in that the lesions have been produced in a primate which, in nutritional metabolism, is closely related to man. Furthermore, the lesions have resulted from an experimental circumstance that might occur in man. Pyridoxine deficiency is, in essence, a chronic deficiency, relatively slow in evolution and without distinctive external manifestations. Such a deficiency state would be one particularly difficult of clinical recognition.

Later in the same article Rinehart and Greenberg hypothesized that the human disease originated in a chronic vitamin B$_6$ deficiency, which led *somehow* to a defect in the metabolism of protein, which in turn could *somehow* produce arterial lesions.

This was obviously a landmark study. The results were published in a leading journal, the *American Journal of Pathology,* and at additional expense because of the color plate. Rinehart was already a noted scientist. He was chairman of the Department of Pathology at the University of California-San Francisco Medical School. A year after the study was published, in 1949, he became president of the American Society for Experimental Pathology. Greenberg was an Assistant Professor of Pathology and Pharmacology at the same university. The year after the article was published, he was promoted to Associate Professor. The team had credibility and distinction, yet the research did not immediately lead to a wave of papers extending the findings by other investigators interested in arteriosclerosis. It was not for lack of confirmation of the work. Within a decade other workers substantiated the results. In the United States, C. W. Mushett and G. Emerson carried out similar experiments in dogs and monkeys, confirming that a pyridoxine-deficient diet caused arteriosclerosis. A Japanese medical group, also using monkeys, again confirmed Rinehart and Greenberg (Kuzuya 1959).

There was, however, a team of dissenting investigators who attempted to reproduce the results of Rinehart and Greenberg without success. This group, from Harvard University, included Dr. Frederick J. Stare and Dr. George V. Mann (whom we quoted earlier). They had conducted a series of dietary cholesterol experiments on monkeys, and remarked in passing that when they kept a rhesus monkey on a vitamin B_6-deficient diet for nine months, they saw no significant gross arterial lesions. Microscopic investigation revealed some lesions that appeared similar to those described by Rinehart and Greenberg, but the lesions were not considered very dramatic or important by the Harvard authors (Mann et al. 1953).

Three years later (1956) in another paper co-authored by Mann, brief mention was again made of negative results obtained when feeding monkeys a diet deficient in vitamin B_6. A future paper was promised dealing specifically with pyridoxine-deficient monkeys and arterial lesions. Such a paper never appeared in print. When we questioned Mann in 1978, he referred us to an article published in 1968. It fell far short of a definitive work. The paper concerned pyridoxine-deficient monkeys who were examined after death brought about by the deficiency. Only one paragraph dealt with vascular pathology. Mann wrote that the monkeys had been eating poorly, and had suffered considerable weight loss. "A notable feature of animals autopsied after death from pyridoxine deficiency was the almost complete absence of body fat in any of the usual depot sites."

And therein lies a clue why he had failed to confirm Rinehart and Greenberg's studies.

When dealing with experimental vitamin B_6 deficiency one must perform a balancing act. If too much vitamin B_6 is given, then little arteriosclerosis will be seen since the animal won't be sufficiently deficient. If the vitamin B_6 deficiency is too severe, however, little arteriosclerosis will develop for another reason. Arteriosclerosis is primarily a disease of abnormal proliferation and growth of smooth muscle cells. For atheromas to develop ("oma" means new tissue), cells must be capable of growing. Drs. Peter Holtz and Dieter Palm of the Pharmaceutical Institute of Frankfurt University in Germany pointed out in 1964 that since vitamin B_6 functions in numerous reactions concerned with the synthesis of amino acids and proteins prerequisites to growth, it was to be expected that a deficiency would lead to inhibition of growth.

Severe enough vitamin B_6 deficiency, especially under a high protein load, leads to weight loss, followed by rapid death. Deficiency studies must provide enough vitamin B_6 for growth of cells in the atheromas, yet be skimpy enough to produce a systematic deficiency. Stare and Mann were probably too conscientious in inducing vitamin B_6 deficiency and this allowed no margin for any growth. Without growth, arteriosclerosis could not develop and confirmation of Rinehart and Greenberg would be impossible.

As far as we can ascertain, no other negative results were communicated or hinted at by any authors during the 1950s and 1960s. It is unclear whether the dearth of papers concerning negative findings was due to lack of enthusiasm for the line of investigation, to the influence of Stare and Mann, or to the reluctance of investigators to publish negative results. For whatever reason, the cholesterol hypothesis remained the guiding principle for arteriosclerosis research, and the promising new discovery generated by Rinehart and Greenberg lay dormant in the literature.

Rinehart died in 1955. Greenberg continued in the Department of Pathology at San Francisco. As a full professor of pathology, he presented papers at international conferences as *the* expert, almost by default (since there were so few working in the same area) on the relationship between arteriosclerosis and vitamin B_6 deficiency. He is today Professor Emeritus at the University of California.

In 1969, at a New York Academy of Sciences symposium on experimental medicine and surgery in primates, one of seven sessions was devoted to experimental cardiovascular studies. Of the eight papers presented in the session, six dealt with experimental arteriosclerosis in primates. Three of these made perfunctory mention of the work of Rinehart and Greenberg, and cited their paper. Yet the references could be attributed more to the demands of scholarly completeness than to enthusiastic recognition of the work's relevance. The papers did not deal with the results in a serious way. None of the researchers even commented on the vitamin work except to note that one of the ways that had been reported to produce arteriosclerosis was by withholding vitamin B_6 from the diet. No one commented on whether Rinehart and Greenberg were right or wrong, quaint or important.

METABOLIC ROLE OF VITAMIN B_6

In the course of their studies Rinehart and Greenberg (1956) had also carried out other biochemical work on pyridoxine. It was known that vitamin B_6 is necessary for facilitating more than 40 chemical reactions in the body. One well-studied set of chemical functions of vitamin B_6 is its role in the metabolism of amino acids.

The principal reaction involves transfer of parts of amino acids known as amine groups (clusters of one nitrogen atom and three hydrogen atoms) from the amino acids to other molecules. Rinehart and Greenberg studied this "transaminase" reaction, as it is called, and measured its rate in "normal" humans. They found that administration of vitamin B_6 in relatively small daily doses of 10 to 15 mg for four to six weeks regularly caused a 30 percent to 100 percent increase of transaminase activity. The result introduced the possibility that vitamin B_6 levels in "normal" humans may be below optimum. However, since the benefit (or cost) of high activity was not known, it could not be established that the normal level was pathologically deficient, only that a higher level of vitamin B_6 could raise the rate of the reaction.

In summary, Rinehart and Greenberg's work showed that experimental vitamin B_6 deficiency caused arteriosclerosis. They also found that supplementing vitamin B_6 in humans leads to more active protein metabolism. This is an important point, as we show in the next chapter.

CLINICAL INDICATIONS OF DEFICIENCY OF VITAMIN B_6

In 1955 Dr. Henry Schroeder, who served on the staff of the Hypertension Division of the Department of Internal Medicine at the Washington University School of Medicine, reflected on the implications of the work of Rinehart and Greenberg. Even if vitamin B_6 deficiency could cause arteriosclerosis under laboratory conditions, he asked, were Americans actually deficient in the vitamin? At first glance this seemed unlikely since he was aware that vitamin B_6 is widely distributed in common foods, including meats, grains, and vegetables.

But, Schroeder found that many of the foods that constitute the bulk of American diets actually have low levels of vitamin B_6 because of the way the foods are processed and cooked. Schroeder found that Americans ingested an insufficient amount of the vitamin during most of the year. (In those days two to three mg/day was suggested as an adequate intake of vitamin B_6.) Schroeder also examined different populations around the world and found that although incidence of arteriosclerosis could not be correlated with the general level of nutrition, it *was* related to the amount of vitamin B_6 in the diet. Schroeder's survey was a tentative but important step in the search for clinical and epidemiological correlations that would test the propositions of Rinehart and Greenberg.

VITAMIN B$_6$ LEVELS IN CORONARY PATIENTS

In 1957 Dr. G. E. Boxer, a New York physician, and his colleagues published a report concerning the serum vitamin B$_6$ levels of heart patients. They reasoned that if vitamin B$_6$ deficiency was clinically significant, then heart attack patients should be more deficient in vitamin B$_6$ than the normal population. His group found that heart patients *do* tend to have lower levels of vitamin B$_6$. Although their sample was too small to draw unequivocal conclusions, the results were suggestive. Boxer also found that many mammals (guinea pigs, rats, rabbits, cats, and dogs) had much higher average concentrations of vitamin B$_6$ in their blood than humans or rhesus monkeys—4 to 20 twenty times higher. Boxer's group also found interesting differences in vitamin B$_6$ levels between age groups and between peoples of different societies. Schoolchildren in New York City tended to have higher vitamin B$_6$ levels than adult New Yorkers. At the same time, children in Cuba, who followed a diet significantly different from that of New York children, had vitamin B$_6$ levels that averaged 50 percent higher than those of children in New York.

Following Boxer's publication, Dr. L.G. Gvozdova, and Russian colleagues, reported in 1966 that the concentration of vitamin B$_6$ in the blood of patients with coronary arteriosclerosis was on the average 4.5 times lower than that of healthy persons. (This study involved 48 patients with arteriosclerosis and 21 healthy people.) The Russian group also confirmed the expectation that supplements of vitamin B$_6$ could raise the blood pyridoxine concentrations of coronary patients to levels equal to or above those of normal patients.

These two studies show that populations can differ significantly in blood levels of vitamin B$_6$. The most compelling finding is that victims of heart attacks are low in vitamin B$_6$. The results, however, have not yet had an impact on clinical approaches to treating arteriosclerosis.

THE CONTRACEPTIVE PILL, VITAMIN B_6 DEFICIENCY, AND ARTERIOSCLEROSIS

Coronary patients are not the only group that have low levels of vitamin B_6. Young healthy women taking oral contraceptives (birth control pills) also tend to be vitamin B_6 deficient. For instance, in 1973 Dr. P. W. Adams and an English team of doctors found that "80 percent of women taking oral contraceptives have abnormal tryptophan [an amino acid] metabolism, indicating a relative vitamin B_6 deficiency and that about 20 percent have evidence of absolute deficiency in this vitamin."

Vitamin B_6 is required to convert tryptophan to several different compounds. The investigators in England had previously established the experimental limits of what they defined as "relative" and "absolute" deficiency by carrying out a set of tests to measure the rates of biochemical reactions that required vitamin B_6 (Rose et al. 1973). If one of the enzymes in the body that depended on vitamin B_6 had an activity that was significantly lower than what was considered normal (below 97.7 percent of the rest of the population), then the woman was considered to have a "relative" deficiency in the vitamin. If two or more of the enzymes measured showed activity that was significantly below normal, then the woman had an "absolute" deficiency in the vitamin.

The investigators found that some women with absolute deficiency also suffered mental depression, consisting of "pessimism, anxiety dissatisfaction, lethargy and loss of libido. . . . Almost every woman complained during the first interview of greater lability of emotions with increased weepiness and irritability." It was found that these women responded to treatment with vitamin B_6 supplements (20 mg twice daily), while those with relative deficiency who were also depressed "showed no such response" to vitamin B_6 supplements.

Although this relationship is interesting, we mention it because of a larger issue: With 80 percent of the users of the contraceptive pill in England shown to be deficient in vitamin

B_6, millions of women have been subjected to an inadvertent experiment in long term vitamin B_6 deficiency. If Rinehart and Greenberg are correct, these women collectively should show signs of advanced cardiovascular pathology. Since arteriosclerosis is a slowly developing disease, only now, after 15 to 20 years of large-scale use of the contraceptive pill, would one expect these effects to be manifest. In fact, such increases in vascular disease in contraceptive pill users are now being reported in the medical literature.

Two studies were published in *The Lancet* on October 8, 1977. One enormous survey, conducted by the Royal College of General Practitioners, involved 46,000 women. Half (23,000) the women in the study were taking the contraceptive pill; they were matched by age and marital status against 23,000 non-Pill-users. The investigators found that

> The death rate in those who had taken the Pill continuously for 5 years or more was 10 times that of the controls. The excess deaths in oral-contraception users were due to a wide range of vascular conditions. The total mortality-rate in women who had ever used the Pill was increased 40 percent and this was due to an increase in deaths from circulatory diseases. . . . The excess was substantially greater than the death rate from complications of pregnancy in the controls and was double the death-rate from accidents. The excess mortality-rate increased with age, cigarette smoking, and duration of oral contraceptive use.

The second study, involving 17,000 women, was undertaken by Dr. M. P. Vessey and a team of physicians at the Department of Social and Community Medicine at Oxford University. These researchers also concluded:

> The cardiovascular risks associated with oral-contraception use in this country are of an appreciable magnitude.

The conclusions of these two studies have been confirmed in the United States by Dr. Hershel Jick and his colleagues of the Boston Collaborative Drug Surveillance Program at Boston

University Medical Center and the Department of Epidemiology, Harvard University School of Public Health. The group found in 1978 that "in otherwise healthy young women the relative risk of myocardial infarction for oral contraceptive users compared to nonusers is estimated to be about 15."

We find it somewhat surprising that none of these studies made mention of any connection between the observed prevalence of cardiovascular disease and the known vitamin B_6 deficiencies of women on the contraceptive pill. But medicine seems sometimes to be a curiously ahistorical profession and the vitamin B_6/oral contraceptive link becomes significant only if one takes seriously the results of Rinehart and Greenberg's work of 20 and 30 years earlier. This work unfortunately belongs to a now rarely examined era.

The recent British and American studies indicate that the increased death rate in oral contraceptive users attributed to vascular disease is related to increased arteriosclerosis. But they do so indirectly, by statistical association. The results of direct study, however, also show that oral contraceptive use promotes arteriosclerosis. In the early 1970s Dr. Nelson Irey and his colleagues at the Armed Forces Institute of Pathology in Washington, D.C., compared arterial tissue of young women who had used oral contraceptives with those who did not. They found that the women using oral contraceptives had "severe intimal proliferation" that resulted in narrowing of the lumen. Irey's group felt the abnormal proliferations were "primary intrinsic vascular alterations" of arteriosclerosis.

So it appears that oral contraceptive use leads to acceleration of the arteriosclerotic process.

VITAMIN B_6 DEFICIENCY AND BLOOD COAGULATION

One of the consequences of arteriosclerosis is a narrowing of the lumen as a result of the proliferation and growth of cells in the arterial walls. Further trouble develops when blood clots develop at the plaques. And now work by Dr. Kuchibhotla Subbarao of Temple University and colleagues has shown that low vitamin B_6 levels increase the tendency for the blood to coagulate. So it appears that high vitamin B_6 plays a double role: preventing both arteriosclerosis and abnormal blood clotting.

The consequences of vitamin B_6 deficiency are sufficiently serious to warrant further work. The current findings are that experimental vitamin B_6 deficiency can lead to arteriosclerosis in monkeys; Americans eat diets that are vitamin B_6 deficient; coronary patients have much lower vitamin B_6 levels than normal people; women taking the birth control pill tend to be vitamin B_6 deficient, and have been proven higher cardiovascular risks; vitamin B_6 deficiency increases blood coagulation. The implications of these findings become even more significant when the results are linked to experimental results described in the next chapter, which show that vitamin B_6 deficiency leads to elevated serum levels of homocysteine.

CHAPTER 4

The Homocysteine Theory

CONCERN WITH HOMOCYSTEINE began with two young sisters, Patricia B. and Pauline B., who lived in Belfast, Northern Ireland, in the early 1960s. They both had thin blond hair and fair skin, not unusual characteristics for Irish girls, but they shared other physical characteristics that made them peculiar. The lenses inside their blue eyes were abnormally situated. Instead of resting in the normal position, the lenses were displaced and loose. Also, every time the girls moved their eyes, their irises quivered. Both girls were knock-kneed and had abnormally high arches in their feet. They walked with a shuffle and had difficulty going up and down stairs. Both had suffered seizures. The girls also were severely retarded. Patricia, age six, had an I.Q. of 30 and Pauline, age four, was not given an I.Q. test because her mental capacity was even lower. Patricia had a working vocabulary of about 12 words. Pauline could not yet speak. Their mother, age 32, was in good general health.

The girls came to the attention of Dr. Claude Field during a medical examination. He took urine samples from the sisters and sent them to Dr. Nina Carson and Dr. D. W. Neill at the Royal Belfast Hospital for Sick Children. Carson and Neill were engaged in a biochemical survey of all mentally retarded persons in Northern Ireland. It was known that in some rare cases, genetic abnormalities of amino acid metabolism lead to mental retardation. Drs. Carson and Neill set out to register those families susceptible to amino acid metabolic disorders since with early enough diagnosis, physicians can sometimes intervene to prevent the retardation.

The screening technique developed by Dr. C. E. Dent and his group at University College Hospital, London, was sufficiently general so that in the course of their work, Carson and Neill discovered an abnormality not previously described. Patricia and Pauline were excreting quantities of a sulfur-containing amino acid not normally seen in urine. The amino acid was recognized by Dr. Roland Westall of Dent's group to be homocystine. Homocystine is, in turn, made up of two identical halves bonded together; each half is called homocysteine. Because the homocystine was found in the urine, Carson and Neill and their London collaborators named the disorder "homocystinuria" ("uria" meaning in the urine; homocystine in the blood is called homocysteinemia). Carson and Neill had in fact discovered a new genetic disease whose most apparent symptom was mental retardation. As we will soon see this disease later provided an immensely valuable clue to understanding arteriosclerosis.

Almost simultaneously, T. Gerritsen and associates at the University of Wisconsin Medical School in Madison, screening children with mental retardation, observed that one patient, a one-year-old infant, excreted homocystine.

The cases of homocystinuria led to expanded clinical interest in the amino acid methionine, which is consumed in food and is processed by the body to make homocystine. Methionine is present in *both* animal and vegetable protein. Once protein is eaten, it is broken down into its amino acid parts by the digestive enzymes in the stomach and intestine. The amino acids are transported into the blood and delivered to individual cells. Most cells of the body are able to carry out subsequent chemical reactions using the amino acids. Biochemical charts have been constructed showing how amino acids are altered by specific enzymes. The metabolism of methionine was well known in 1962, when Pauline and Patricia were being studied. The chart on the following page shows how methionine is changed in the cells of the body.

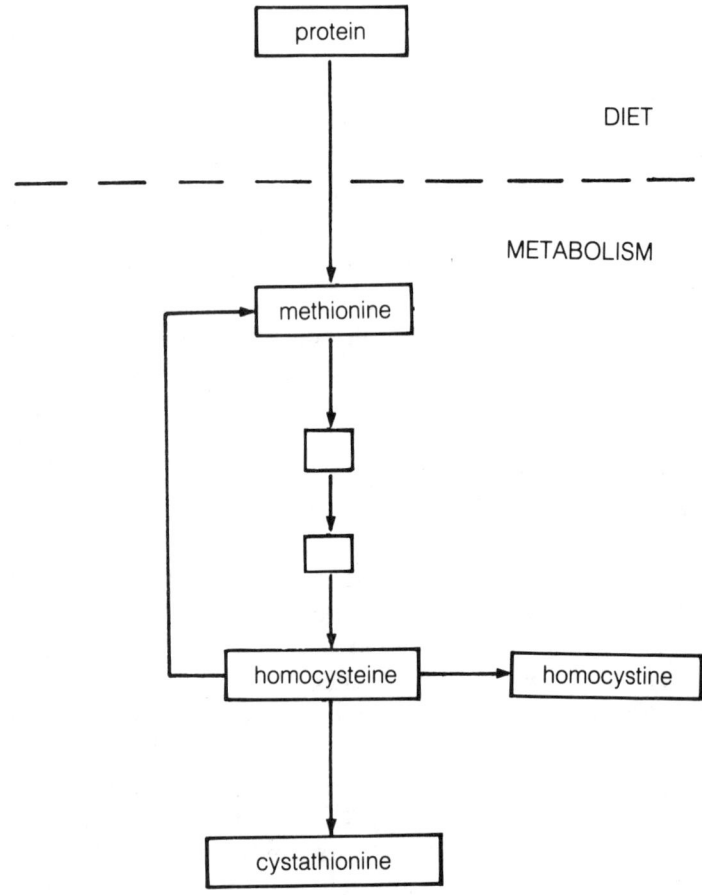

This biochemical chart shows how the body metabolizes the amino acid methionine to homocysteine and related compounds. Each step involves an enzyme. Homocysteine can be converted to cystathionine or reconverted to methionine. If homocysteine is at abnormally high levels, some of it will be converted to homocystine and excreted in the urine.

A similar chart appeared in Carson's study in 1963 where she discussed the metabolic consequences of homocystinuria.

Molecules are altered by enzymes, which add or remove one chemical subunit at each step. In the chart we can see that methionine is transformed to homocysteine through two stages, here represented by empty boxes. Homocysteine is then either converted to cystathionine (by the enzyme cystathionine synthase) or it is recovered as methionine. These details may seem very technical, but, as we will show shortly, they are, indeed, important. Normal humans contain a small amount of methionine and a very small amount of homocysteine in their blood. Because of a metabolic abnormality, however, people with the disease homocystinuria have much larger than normal amounts of homocysteine in the blood. Some homocysteine is converted to homocystine, and is then excreted in the urine.

Dr. Carson and her colleagues in Belfast, along with Dent and his colleagues from University College Hospital in London, carefully studied Patricia and Pauline. They found there was a complete metabolic block at the step where homocysteine is converted to cystathionine. Thus, homocysteine and methionine built up to the point where the body excreted them in large quantities in the urine.

HOMOCYSTINURIA AND VASCULAR DISEASE

Carson and colleagues pursued the pathology of the disease. They reported on four children who had earlier been screened for homocystinuria and had subsequently died (Gibson et al. 1964). All were surprisingly young, ranging in age (at death) from 7 to 13 years. One was Patricia who died at age 9½. She had been operated on two weeks previously to remove her defective lenses. She was making an apparently normal recovery when she died of a massive coronary.

It was immediately evident in doing the autopsies that all the children, including Patricia (whose autopsy had been done by Dr. A. T. Edwards and Dr. Gerald Gaull), had extensive abnormalities of their blood vessels. "The most striking lesions were vascular." The researchers found fibrous thickenings of the intima, and prominent and irregular internal elastic lamina. They also found a prevalence of thromboses (Carson et al. 1965). It was as if the whole arteriosclerotic process, which usually takes decades to develop, had occurred at a much accelerated pace. This suggested a link between homocystine and arteriosclerosis (although in published reports the word "arteriosclerosis" is not used), at least in this small group.

Other work confirmed the link. In 1965 Dr. Neil Schimke and his colleagues at Johns Hopkins University screened a population for homocystinuria by checking ophthalmological patients who had displaced lenses. The original connection between displaced lenses and homocystinuria had been made in Patricia and Pauline, and Schimke's group found that of those with displaced lenses, 5 percent had homocystinuria. They studied 20 families of homocystinurics and found 38 affected members. Records showed that 10 percent of these people died extremely early, at ages ranging between 3 and 28. *All had died of vascularly related causes, particularly thrombotic occlusion associated with thickened arterial intima.* A majority of the patients were mentally retarded but 16 of the 38 had normal intelligence.

Research on homocystinuria served to establish the association between homocystine and arteriosclerosis, but it did not explain the connection, and it might seem we have strayed from our direct concern with arteriosclerosis in the general population. Not entirely, as we shall show.

Vascular specialists, learning of the new disease, might well have made a mental note. But the disease is rare as well as novel, affecting only about one in 80,000 people. It was an additional piece in a puzzle that was already complex and confusing. The disease was also associated with other features, such as mental retardation and ophthalmological defects, which bore no discernible relation to arteriosclerosis in normal people. Vascular specialists could understandably view homocystinuria as a quite peripheral clue to the cure of arteriosclerosis, a disease affecting a majority of the population.

Other physicians, however, were concerned with therapy for homocystinuria and this led them to vitamin B₆.

HOMOCYSTEINE AND VITAMIN B$_6$

In 1965 Drs. George Spaeth and G. Winston Barber of the Willis Eye Hospital in Philadelphia recalled an important biochemical fact that had been omitted from the charts of methionine metabolism published by Carson and, later, Schimke. In order to transform homocysteine to cystathionine, the enzyme cystathionine synthase is necessary—but so is a co-enzyme (a small molecule that must be present before certain biochemical reactions can take place). This co-enzyme is vitamin B$_6$! Spaeth and Barber suggested that homocystinurics might reduce their serum homocysteine levels with high doses of vitamin B$_6$. They tried just such therapy with a homo-cystinuric patient to see if there would be any improvement in his condition. There was "slight normalization: decrease in urinary homocystine, increase in cystine and cystathionine." The vitamin therapy was modestly effective and led to a modest proposition: Perhaps the enzyme cystathionine synthase is present in abnormal form, unable to react properly with its co-enzyme.

These results were not particularly conclusive but vitamin B$_6$ became of immediate interest. In the next four years, others, including Carson in Belfast and Gaull in New York, investigated the use of vitamin B$_6$ therapy for homocystinurics. It has turned out that homocystinuria is not one disease, but a syndrome of at least two distinct illnesses. In one set of cases, which represents approximately half the patients with the disease, vitamin B$_6$ therapy leads to an almost complete disappearance of homocys-teine from the blood and the return to normal levels of methionine. The other set of patients apparently cannot utilize the vitamin B$_6$, and for them no substantive changes occur.

Spaeth and Barber's paper shows that even equivocal journal results can be seminal. Their proposal of vitamin B$_6$ therapy for homocystinuria produced striking results in other clinics and

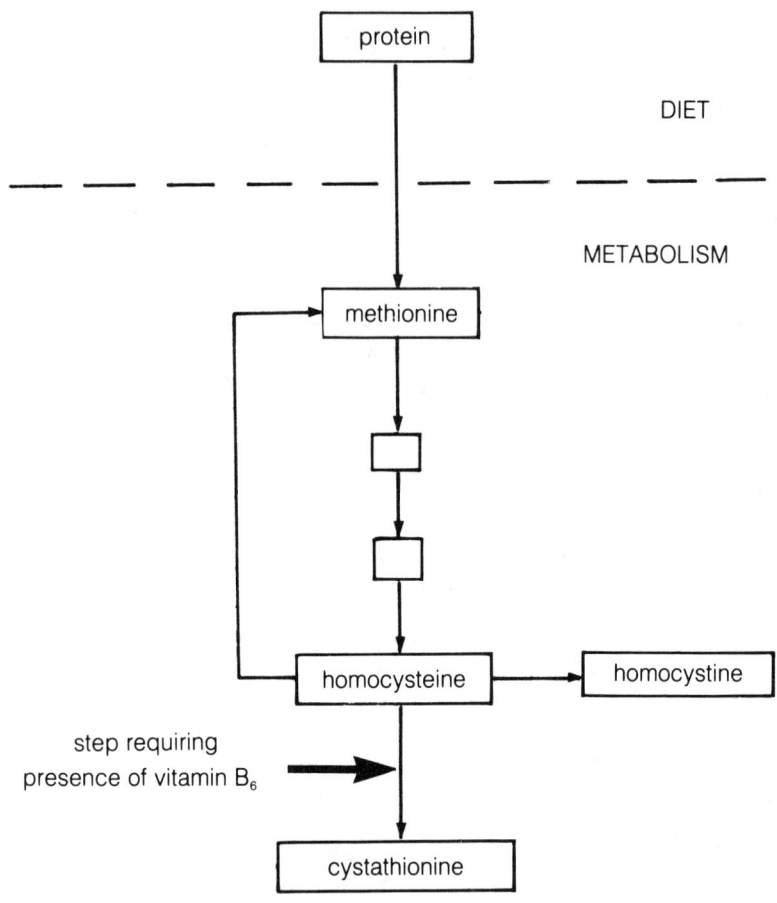

The same biochemical chart of methionine metabolism as on p. 70, but also showing relationship of vitamin B_6 to homocysteine. If there is insufficient B_6, the step converting homocysteine to cystathionine cannot take place and homocystine will accumulate in the body.

eventually in theirs also, when used on the appropriate patients.

THE CAUSE OF ARTERIOSCLEROSIS

Work on vitamin B_6 and work on homocysteine metabolism thus converged in the late 1960s. There was still no obvious experimental relationship between these compounds and the underlying cause of arteriosclerosis. But the foundations had been laid. What was needed was an individual in the right place with the right training and a willingness to consider bold revisions of existing ideas.

Dr. Kilmer McCully was a pathologist on the faculty of the Harvard Medical School and the Massachusetts General Hospital. He had developed an interest in the problem of arteriosclerosis while still in medical school, and was a student at Harvard when Drs. Stare and Mann conducted their work on cholesterol (and vitamin B_6 deficiency) in monkeys. He was familiar with the results of these experiments and had pondered their implications. After medical school, McCully spent several years working in biochemistry and learning biochemical techniques. He worked in the laboratories of Dr. James Watson (co-discoverer of the structure of DNA) and Dr. Konrad Bloch (discoverer of the steps in the biosynthesis of cholesterol), both of whom received the Nobel Prize for their work. After these research positions McCully completed his three-year residence in pathology. Later, he met Dr. Mary Efron at the Massachusetts General Hospital. She had worked with Dr. C. E. Dent in London before heading a research group concerned with abnormalities of amino acid metabolism. She was curious about the underlying pathologies associated with such diseases. Dr. Efron referred McCully to two patients who had died from effects related to homocystinuria. She suggested that the underlying pathology might be worth examining. McCully's investigations showed that both patients had arteriosclerosis. One, a male infant, who died at only seven and a half weeks, could not reconvert homocysteine back to methionine. He had had homocystinuria. The other patient, who died at age eight, was mentally retarded, and apparently had homocystinuria caused by cystathionine synthase deficiency.

In 1969 McCully reported in the *American Journal of Pathology* that both patients had numerous lesions in various sized arteries. "The lumens of many large and medium-sized arteries were narrowed by . . . fibrosis." The eight-year-old had developed more advanced lesions but the pattern of the arteriosclerosis was clear in both. One patient had high methionine, high homocystine, and low cystathionine; the other patient had low methionine, high homocystine, and high cystathionine. High homocystine levels seemed to be the culprit since homocystine was the only amino acid with a raised concentration in both patients.

McCully had studied the work of Rinehart and Greenberg on production of arteriosclerosis by vitamin B_6 deficiency, as well as the recent reports on homocystinuria. He was familiar with the connection between vitamin B_6 and homocysteine metabolism. In his paper describing the vascular pathology of the homocystinuric patients, McCully went much further by proposing a new explanation for arteriosclerosis itself.

Is it possible . . . that in patients with hereditary, dietary, environmental or other predisposition to arteriosclerosis—such as that observed in those who have diabetes, hypothyroidism, hypertension, radiation injury, or who smoke cigarettes—vascular damage and fibrous arterial plaques develop as a result of elevated concentrations of homocysteine or . . . derivatives? Although the current emphasis in the field of pathogenesis of arteriosclerosis is on the importance of dietary fat and the stability of the various plasma lipid fractions on the development of lipid plaques and the conversion of fibrous plaques to lipid plaques, considerable opinion and evidence can be found in the literature that vascular damage, similar to that found in these patients with homocysteinemia, is the initial pathogenic factor in arteriosclerosis, and that lipid deposition is a secondary complication of the primary vascular alteration. . . . The puzzling observation that pyridoxine-deficient monkeys develop arteriosclerotic lesions can be explained by assuming that an elevated homocysteine concentration produced by pyridoxine deficiency led to initial vascular damage in these animals. . . . The metabolic effects of homocysteine that lead to arterial damage are obscure, and the observations presented in this report suggest a promising area for future research in the pathogenesis of arteriosclerosis.

We call McCully's new explanation of the cause of arteriosclerosis the homocysteine theory, and it leads to several testable predictions.

(1) Homocysteine should induce arteriosclerosis in animals on an experimental basis.

(2) People with vitamin B_6 deficiency should accumulate higher levels of homocysteine in their blood and thus be susceptible to arteriosclerosis.

(3) People having arteriosclerosis, such as coronary patients, should tend to have higher levels of homocysteine in their blood.

Each of these propositions has been verified.

INDUCTION OF ARTERIOSCLEROSIS BY HOMOCYSTEINE

Does homocysteine cause arteriosclerosis? McCully, together with Dr. Bruce Ragsdale, tested this proposition in 1970. They divided 24 rabbits into eight groups. Some were given injections of homocysteine. Others were given diets that were normal, and still others were given diets deficient in vitamin B_6 or supplemented with cholesterol. After 35 days, the researchers found that all the animals given homocysteine and all the animals given a vitamin B_6-deficient diet showed "early fibrous arteriosclerotic plaques, both in the [aortic] arch and in the abdominal aorta." Five of the homocysteine-injected animals showed more severe pathology; the aortas were thickened and lesions were found. Only one of six controls on the normal diet and one of three animals on the cholesterol diet showed fibrous arteriosclerotic plaques.

McCully and Ragsdale concluded that "the experimental lesions reproduce the essential features of the vascular pathology associated with [high homocysteine levels in the blood]. . . . Furthermore, the distribution of the experimental lesions . . . as well as the [tissue] changes, are characteristic of the early fibrous plaques encountered in human arteriosclerosis."

The homocysteine theory looked promising and McCully and Ragsdale discussed some of its implications. Their results were in accord with Rinehart and Greenberg's observations of atherosclerosis in vitamin B_6-deficient primates. The results also supported McCully's earlier idea that an elevated homocysteine level due to vitamin B_6 deficiency produced arterial lesions. The investigators also suggested that high methionine diets might lead to arteriosclerosis in laboratory animals, as well as in humans, since these diets might result in elevated homocysteine synthesis. Finally, they voiced the possibility that many of the known risk factors might cause arteriosclerosis indirectly as a consequence of influencing homocysteine metabolism.

The first research group that attempted to confirm McCully and Ragsdale's work failed to demonstrate a conclusive effect of homocysteine. Dr. Sheila Donahue, Dr. Gerald Gaull, and colleagues at the New York State Institute for Basic Research in Mental Retardation and the Mount Sinai School of Medicine (1974) repeated some of the experiments, also using rabbits. Donahue's group injected a solution of a homocysteine compound into weanling rabbits daily for 35 days. Only one hour after an injection they could no longer detect any homocysteine in blood samples taken from the animals. Further, microscopic examination showed no difference between the arteries of experimental and control animals. Donahue and the New York State group interpreted their results as contradicting McCully's work.

There was no obvious way to reconcile McCully and Ragsdale's work with that of Donahue's group. The proposition that homocysteine can cause arteriosclerosis could not be considered strongly established with such a pair of opposite findings.

At that point another group reported significant new findings. Dr. Laurence Harker and a team of investigators in Seattle (1974) used a different method—intravenous infusion—to insure the presence of homocystine in the blood of baboons. They thereby created sustained homocystinemia. The concentration of homocystine was similar to that found in the blood of homocystinuric patients. They showed that under this condition homocystine rapidly caused extensive signs of arteriosclerosis. They observed that the inner layer of endothelial cells within the artery was dramatically destroyed. After a week of induced homocystinemia, 23 percent of the endothelium was lost. In animals given even higher doses of homocystine, about two to five times that of human homocystinurics, arterial occlusion developed within a week.

The Harker team study was an important addition to the homocysteine literature. It was very conservatively written, with an emphasis on blood clot formation and homocystinemia, and did not deal with the larger question of arteriosclerosis in the general population. Nonetheless, the study confirmed the first tenet of the homocysteine theory—arteriosclerosis can be induced with homocystine.

In a larger study in 1976 the same group extended their findings that experimental homocystinemia caused loss of the endothelial lining of arteries. They found that the higher the level of homocystine, the more severely injured the inner arterial surface. Equally important, they found a 15-fold increase in cell division in the arterial endothelium at the higher levels of homocystine.

On the other hand, cholesterol levels found in the blood were not correlated with either the lesions or the proliferation of the endothelium. The authors summarized their interpretation in an exquisitely diplomatic paragraph worded to avoid stepping on the toes of those immersed in the cholesterol hypothesis:

Although we find no evidence to implicate hypercholesterolemia or hypertriglyceridemia in homocystine-induced vascular injury, the importance of lipids in the genesis of atherosclerosis has long been emphasized but poorly understood. Clearly, lipid accumulation both within the smooth muscle cells and in the surrounding matrix is important in preventing lesion regression. . . . Of equal interest are observations suggesting that chronic (9 months or longer) sustained hypercholesterolemia will result in endothelia "injury" and focal denudation similar to that observed in the homocystinemic animals in the present study. Thus lipids may exert in part a similar effect to that seen in homocystinemia.

Translated: Homocystine rapidly induces the initial stages of arteriosclerosis and cholesterol effects are not apparent. Cholesterol may have a role in maintaining lesions or perhaps may be a secondary cause. The researchers made no direct mention of McCully's theory, but of necessity they made reference to his articles and were obviously influenced by his work. However, they did not discuss or even ask a key question suggested by their study—could there be elevated homocystine levels in "normal" people owing, perhaps, to some dietary deficiency such as vitamin B_6? In fact, earlier work had already explored this issue.

VITAMIN B_6 DEFICIENCY AND HOMOCYSTINURIA

In 1970, Y. Park and Hellen Linkswiler of the Department of Nutritional Science at the University of Wisconsin studied the relationship between low vitamin B_6 diets and metabolism of methionine. They gave six male subjects an experimental diet that was high in protein and low in vitamin B_6 (0.16 mg/day). Although the diet contained high amounts of protein (150 gm per day in the form of casein and gelatin), it also contained peaches, pears, grapefruit juice, carrots, celery, and onions. In essence, this was no more peculiar than the diet of people who subsist on coffee and fast foods. For the initial 14 days of the experiment the subjects were given dietary supplements of vitamin B_6 (2 mg/day). They were then maintained on the experimental diet alone without vitamin B_6 supplements.

Prior to vitamin B_6 depletion, Park and Linkswiler found no homocystine in the urine of subjects. On the seventh day of the low vitamin B_6 diet, the subjects were given a dose of methionine to trace its conversion into other molecules. Unlike subjects with sufficient vitamin B_6, a trace amount of homocystine could be detected in the urine of two of the six subjects. By the 21st day all six subjects maintained on the vitamin B_6-deficient diet excreted substantial amounts of homocystine after being given methionine. In addition, by the 21st day, trace amounts of homocystine began to appear in the urine of three of the six subjects even *before* receiving methionine. Following the 21-day period, the subjects were again given daily vitamin B_6 supplements (2 mg/day). Homocystine levels declined dramatically, though one subject continued to excrete detectable amounts of homocystine for one week.

Park and Linkswiler's study showed that vitamin B_6 deficiency alone can lead to abnormal amounts of homocystine. It thus provides experimental evidence for the second prediction of the homocysteine theory: People with vitamin B_6 deficiency should accumulate higher levels of homocysteine in their blood.

CORONARY PATIENTS AND HOMOCYSTINEMIA

In 1976 the *Journal of Clinical Investigation* published a study by Drs. David and Bridget Wilcken of the Department of Medicine, Prince Henry Hospital and the Oliver Latham Laboratory of Sydney, Australia. "We undertook the present study [they wrote] to explore the possibility that premature coronary artery disease [in patients under 50] is associated with methionine metabolism."

The Wilckens worked with a group of 25 male patients who had severe arteriosclerotic obstructions amounting to a 70 percent block of one or more major branches of a coronary artery. Twenty-two normal people served as non-arteriosclerotic controls. (Seventeen of the normal people were clear of major arterial obstruction.) The other five controls were healthy volunteers presumed normal without testing. The homocysteine levels in both groups were measured after the patients drank a morning glass of orange juice containing a significant but not an enormous amount of methionine, corresponding roughly to that found in 1½ pounds of lean round beef. The serum levels of methionine, homocysteine, and cysteine were measured and compared to a sample taken before the dose of methionine.

The Wilckens' results showed that the arteriosclerotic group had higher cysteine and homocysteine levels. By the tests used, cysteine and homocysteine could be detected in only five of the 22 controls, but they appeared in the serum samples of 17 of the 25 coronary patients. Furthermore, seven members of the arteriosclerotic group were in this high cysteine-homocysteine bracket, whereas only one of the controls had high levels. And so the third prediction of the homocysteine theory—that patients suffering arteriosclerosis have higher homocysteine levels—was verified.

The Wilckens were primarily interested in clinically useful findings. They expressed dismay at the prevailing concept of arteriosclerosis. "It is not uncommon for individual patients to have a paucity, or complete absence, of known risk factors, a finding more readily apparent to the practicing physician than to the epidemiologist."

SUMMARY OF THE HOMOCYSTEINE THEORY

The homocysteine theory states that two dietary factors operate in tandem to cause arteriosclerosis in humans. One is consumption of a particular constituent of protein, methionine. The other factor is vitamin B_6 deficiency. If methionine consumption is high and vitamin B_6 intake is too low, homocysteine builds up. Homocysteine induces arteriosclerotic plaques in the cellular lining of blood vessels. An elevated homocysteine level, however it is produced, is the final common pathway for generation of arteriosclerosis.

THE NATURE OF THE PLAQUES

How can homocysteine cause changes in the walls of arteries?

To start with, we know that arteriosclerosis begins with the proliferation of smooth muscle cells in the intimal layer. Drs. Earl and John Benditt (1973) of the University of Washington School of Medicine found that there is something unusual about these proliferating cells. They investigated whether the smooth muscle cells in an atheroma were derived from many cells or from a single one. In other words, they checked to see if many cells independently start to divide or if one cell proliferates into a clone.

The Benditts studied certain "heterozygotic" women who had died of various causes. These women have cells in their bodies that can be chemically distinguished into two groups, type A and type B. When the Benditts looked at aortic patches that were free of arteriosclerotic plaques, they found a mosaic of both type A cells and type B cells. However, when they looked at small atheromas, they found that some plaques had type A cells and other plaques had type B cells, but individual plaques did not contain both type A cells and type B cells. This implied that single plaques were derived from single cells. Otherwise, if many cells had initially divided, then redivided, both type A cells and type B cells would have been found. The result indicates that homocysteine need act on only a single cell in order to start an atheroma.

HOW NORMAL CELLS GROW

The cells in the plaques studied by the Benditts were of course abnormal. If one takes some normal cells, say skin cells, and places them in a petri dish (a shallow laboratory dish) containing water and nutrients, the cells will continue to live and grow and divide. In relatively short order, they will spread out over the entire dish, forming a single layer. At that point, they will stop dividing. It is believed that a substance on the surface of cells can detect the presence of adjacent cells. By some unknown mechanism when cells contact, they inhibit each other from further growth and division, a phenomenon called "contact inhibition."

EFFECT OF HOMOCYSTEINE ON CELL GROWTH

Kilmer McCully studied how homocysteine affects the growth and multiplication of cells. He found that skin cells grown in petri dishes produced a kind of long fibrous molecule known as a *proteoglycan* (because it is made of protein and sugar; "glycan" means sugar). When he added homocysteine to the cells, they produced abnormal looking proteoglycans that were granular in appearance and had a higher sulfur content (remember, homocysteine is a sulfur-containing amino acid). The homocysteine-fed cells also grew in an abnormal way: instead of forming a uniform single layer of cells, there were "areas of growth in which cells formed multiple layers," McCully noted. In the presence of homocysteine there was thus a reduction in contact inhibition, which led to the plaquelike condition of multiple cell layers. McCully also showed that the homocysteine is converted into a related compound, *homocysteic acid* (which, like homocysteine, contains sulfur). This molecule acts as a growth agent and cell toxin.

IMPLICATIONS

In the walls of arteries homocysteine (or a chemical derivative) apparently acts on cells in the same way as it does in the petri dish. It seems to prevent contact inhibition. This could lead to decoupling of cells of the endothelial lining, leaving gaps so that the cells no longer act as a protective sheath, and thus exposing the deeper layers of the arterial wall to the blood. In addition, homocysteine or a derivative, such as homocysteic acid, seems to cause smooth cells to grow abnormally and start piling up on each other.

We do not yet know how a particular cell becomes the progenitor of a clone by transforming into a rapidly dividing entity leading to an atheroma. One reasonable possibility is that homocysteine acts as the transforming agent. This still must be tested, but in any case, homocysteine and its derivatives can certainly facilitate the growth of new cells once the process starts. Dr. Laurence Harker and his colleagues think that a factor in blood platelets (cells that help form clots) may cause smooth muscle cells to divide. Harker has shown that homocystine causes the loss of the cells of the endothelial lining, which normally acts as a barrier between the blood and the rest of the arterial wall. Once the barrier is breached the platelet factor can reach further in.

Recently the toxic effects of the homocysteine derivative homocysteic acid have been studied in nerve cells. Each cell in the body maintains an electrical voltage between the inside and outside of the cell. Homocysteic acid lowers this voltage. The cell attempts to restore the voltage, requiring a great increase in energy and, for reasons that are still obscure, the cell eventually dies. It is possible that the endothelial cells of the blood vessels are killed in the same way.

Obviously much remains to be explored. But the initial studies exploring the cellular basis of the homocysteine theory have been conducted. The results of the investigations of homocysteine on cell cultures reinforce the desire to see that little homocysteine lingers in the blood.

HOW THE THEORY MAY BE WRONG

Many of the investigators whose work we cite in this chapter might feel we have overstated the homocysteine theory. Therefore, having shown how the theory can explain many aspects of the development of arteriosclerosis, let us pause to look at ways in which we may be wrong. First, the theory may not apply as generally as we have outlined. It is possible that homocystinurics (because of their high serum homocysteine levels) will be the sole victims affected by the amino acid in any clinically significant way.

It is also possible that homocystinuria is only *associated* with arteriosclerosis and is not a pivotal step in the production of the disease. Our earlier arguments against the cholesterol theory can cut both ways.

The disease may indeed have many independent causes, to which homocysteine makes a minor contribution. What has been called arteriosclerosis might turn out to be several arterial diseases; homocysteine could be a crucial factor in one of these diseases. Other arteriosclerotic diseases might have other crucial factors. There are, for example, several distinct types of influenza. Even homocystinuria is not a single disease but a set of diseases.

There are other theories of the origin of arteriosclerosis, which propose that vitamin B_6 deficiency is crucial but not because of its relation to homocysteine. These theories implicate other processes dependent on vitamin B_6. Dr. Charles Levene (1978) of the University of Cambridge, England, suggests that vitamin B_6 deficiency leads to improper formation of protein structures of the arterial wall. This causes damage to various elements, including the internal elastic lamina. Dr. David Horrobin and colleagues (1979) at the Clinical Research Institute of Montreal suggest that in the absence of vitamin B_6 the body does not produce enough of a certain fatty acid, prostaglandin E1. The lack of prostaglandin E1 leads to malfunction of certain lymphocytes and other cells, which could affect the arterial wall and result in arteriosclerosis. Both theories are still being developed. They may prove alternatives to the homocysteine theory or they may fit into it in some way.

CRITICISMS

The homocysteine theory has recently generated a wide range of comments and questions.

• A skeptical biochemist dismissed the possibility of people becoming vitamin B_6 deficient, pointing out that bacteria of the human intestinal tract synthesize abundant amounts of the vitamin.

True, our intestinal bacteria do produce vitamin B_6, but they are not a sufficient source. As we described earlier, it is quite simple to make people vitamin-B_6-deficient merely by depriving them of dietary sources of the vitamin. We know that they are deficient because there are drastic changes in the serum concentrations of compounds dependent on the presence of vitamin B_6, including, of course, homocysteine. When these people are fed vitamin B_6 again, the concentrations of vitamin B_6-dependent compounds return to normal.

• An epidemiologist has found fault with all the large epidemiological studies that showed no relationship between diet and serum cholesterol. He suggested that the absence of correlation is due to uncertainty ("slop") in the way data was collected. He suggested that there is indeed a linear relationship between diet and serum cholesterol, but that currently available studies obscure it statistically. So it is not necessary to discard the cholesterol hypothesis for any other theory.

We are perhaps less critical of epidemiological evidence than an epidemiologist would be. But it is striking that the epidemiological record is so unanimous in its findings. These tests were done independently by people favorably disposed to the cholesterol hypothesis. We can assume that these scientists ran the gamut from careful and bright to sloppy and dull, yet their results still agreed.

Even if we suppose that there really is a linear relationship between the amount of cholesterol in one's diet and the amount of cholesterol in one's serum, we may not be able to sustain the cholesterol hypothesis. An individual who is a member of a group that is relatively free of arteriosclerosis (such as the Tukisenta) and who eats very little cholesterol will have serum cholesterol of around 150 mg percent. Let us say that this person then consumes a moderate amount of cholesterol for a few months and his serum cholesterol goes up 10 percent and reaches a plateau. (If you remember when this was tried with the Tukisenta, there was essentially no change in serum cholesterol, but we will disregard that for the purposes of the argument.) Let us subsequently give the individual a larger intake of cholesterol—say, twice that of his moderate dose, which is equal to the intake of the average American. Let us suppose that the individual's serum cholesterol is now 20 percent above his original serum cholesterol level. We can thus say that there is a linear relationship between diet and serum cholesterol. But someone whose serum cholesterol is 180 mg percent does not have high serum cholesterol and is not at high risk. And no clinicians claim to be able to raise or lower the average person's serum cholesterol by more than 20 percent. (There are exceptions to the 20 percent rule but they are few compared to the vast numbers of people that die of the effects of arteriosclerosis.) And this small rise cannot account for the arteriosclerosis in the population, as viewed by the advocates of the cholesterol hypothesis.

• Some investigators suggest that all human beings develop about the same amount of arteriosclerosis. The societies that show few acute signs of the disease, they argue, are those whose members exercise extensively.

The only problem with this suggestion is that it contradicts studies in places such as Israel, where different ethnic groups, examined by the same people, clearly have differing degrees of arteriosclerosis. The Bedouins tend to have thin arterial walls, whereas the Ashkenazi Jews have disease-thickened walls. We will discuss the effects of exercise in the next chapter.

• Couldn't the difference between the Ashkenazi Jews and Bedouins be merely genetic?

As we pointed out in Chapter 1, studies show that when the same genetic population moves to a new environmental setting, it can have a very different rate of coronary heart disease. There may well be a genetic component in arteriosclerosis, and some families could indeed be more susceptible to the disease than other families, but this is no different from the situation in which a whole population is exposed to tuberculosis yet only more susceptible people contract the disease. We know from experience that we can prevent tuberculosis in a population despite a higher susceptibility for the disease by some of its members.

• One molecular biologist has argued that the whole theory is tenuous. Just because coronary patients tend to have low serum vitamin B_6 and high serum homocysteine doesn't mean that much, he insists. Nothing has been proven.

Yes and no. The case is not open and shut. Work remains to be done. But in addition to the clinical observations, direct animal experiments have demonstrated that arteriosclerosis can be induced either by low vitamin B_6 diets or with homocysteine. In addition, the population of North America and Western Europe, where the incidence of arteriosclerosis is high, tends to have a diet that is low in vitamin B_6 and high in methionine.

• Finally, it has been pointed out that in those experiments in which arteriosclerosis was induced by homocysteine, the experimenters used large amounts of homocysteine. How do we know whether lower levels, levels such as those found in people marginally deficient in vitamin B_6, are toxic?

We don't know. The toxicity of homocysteine is increased by increasing its concentration. Since arteriosclerosis is slow to develop, high homocysteine concentrations have been a necessary feature of the experiments testing its effects. There is no quick way to determine if lower homocysteine levels are equally toxic over the long run. That is why the theory is a theory.

But we see the theory as plausible and internally consistent. We feel it should be tested seriously and hope it will be approached with skepticism, but within limits short of nihilistic dismissal of a new idea.

We are left with some puzzles. We do not yet know if dietary methionine, in conjunction with vitamin B_6 deficiency, directly produces arteriosclerosis in humans. It remains to be firmly established that vitamin B_6 exerts a beneficial effect on arteriosclerosis. More experimentation is required to test the theory and encourage the development of effective treatment for cardiovascular disease. It is clear, however, that homocysteine and vitamin B_6 are somehow involved with the disease.

We are impressed with how much the homocysteine theory explains. Homocystinurics have severe arteriosclerosis very early in their lives. Homocystine induces arteriosclerosis in primates in laboratory experiments. People with coronaries tend to have higher serum levels of homocysteine and are deficient in vitamin B_6. As we document in a later chapter, Americans tend to be deficient in vitamin B_6 and to eat large quantities of methionine-containing protein. The theory accounts for much about arteriosclerosis.

In the second part of our book, we start with the working assumption that the homocysteine theory is correct. We will use the theory to tie together many of the risk factors that have been linked to the disease. We will discuss the dietary implications of the theory and develop a new criterion for assessing foods we eat. Finally, we will propose new ways to test the theory and discuss how medical theories come to be accepted.

Part II
Implications of the Theory

CHAPTER 5
Risk Factors

Lagos kills a consul about every two years. The only way to remedy it would be to sleep for the first year on board a ship, or still better, a large hulk anchored off the town in mid-channel. At night the malarious vapour is condensed and concentrated by the chilliness of the ground, and is absorbed or rendered innocuous by passing over a sheet of water.

> *Sir Richard Burton*
> *Abeokuta and the Camaroons Mountains, 1863*

At the time Sir Richard was writing, there were only vague ideas about the nature of malaria. Burton's opinions about the disease were formed by long personal experience in the tropics. It was clear to him that a variety of factors could increase the risk of contracting malaria; he knew that there was something in the air that was more dangerous at night, that the risk was heightened by the chilliness of the ground, and that it was better to sleep in the middle of Lagos Harbor isolated from the shore by moving water.

Cases of malaria were usually contracted near marshy areas, in Africa, of course, but also in other places such as Rome. Many thought the disease came from the air. The English word *malaria* is derived from the Italian *mal' aria*, or "bad air." European scientists suspected vegetable spores and different strains of bacteria as possible causes, but nothing conclusive could be proven. Others believed malaria came from the water. In medical experiments in Italy volunteers drank marsh water or had it injected as an enema or nasal spray. None caught malaria. Leading pathologists studied the blood of malaria victims for many years; then in 1880, Charles Louis Alphonse Laveran finally discovered the malaria parasite. It was not clear, however, how the parasite infected its victims. A Scotsman, Patrick Manson, found that the parasite was also in the mosquito of the genus *Anopheles*, which thus seemed to be a possible carrier of the disease. The problem was that the mosquito sucked the blood of its victims, it didn't appear to pump material the other way. Thus, it seemed unlikely that the mosquito could be the carrier of the parasite.

In 1892, Ronald Ross, an army surgeon in the Indian Medical Service, went to Calcutta and studied bird malaria. Ross found that *Culex* mosquitos feed on sparrows, just as *Anopheles* mosquitos feed on humans. In July 1898 he made the canonical discovery that *Culex* mosquitos pick up the malarial parasite when they bite infected birds and transmit the parasite to uninfected birds, which then become malarious. For this discovery Ross won the Nobel Prize. It turns out that mosquitos not only suck blood from their victims, but they also inject small quantities of anticoagulant to aid in the ingestion of the blood. The malarial parasite is injected with the anticoagulant into the victim (Russell et al. 1963).

Later, investigators showed that the *Anopheles* mosquito transmits malaria to humans in the same way. Its habits became the subject of intense scrutiny. Soon it was learned that the adult is nocturnal and breeds only in standing water. Airborne, the mosquito seldom has an effective range greater than a mile from its breeding pool.

In retrospect, some of Burton's earlier observations make sense. Malaria is a disease of the night because the *Anopheles* is a nocturnal mosquito. The disease is indeed airborne (although not as a vapor). Since malarial mosquitos have a limited range, one would be better off remaining on the moving estuarial water found in Lagos Harbor, far from the stagnant breeding ponds. But the chilliness of the ground has no bearing. It was correlated with the coolness of the night but not causal itself. In fact, at a low enough temperature the ground would become so chilly no mosquito would venture out.

Burton also implied that there was an adaptation period for becoming immune: if a consul could only get beyond the first year uninfected he would survive. This is wrong, yet would be a reasonable expectation on the basis of other infectious diseases, such as measles, where immunity develops after exposure. There was some wisdom in Burton's observations. Yet following all his recommendations would have only slightly enhanced protection. And he did not point the way to a cure.

THE PROBLEM OF VIEWPOINT

Prior to Ross's work, the nineteenth-century view of malaria was that the disease resulted from a complex of factors. Physicians found the various factors difficult to fit together (see diagram). Was it the water or the air temperature that rendered the "malarious vapour" inactive? How did sleeping in mid-channel, far from the swamps, make the malarious vapor less effective? And why did chewing the bark of the cinchona tree ameliorate malarial symptoms?

Ross provided the pivotal insight that revealed the causal relationships of the factors. His discovery that a particular species of nocturnal mosquito transmitted the blood-borne parasite provided a structure to the logical puzzle. Fitting in the other pertinent pieces then became possible.

Discovery of the underlying mechanism of malaria permitted the construction of a model of the disease. The model showed the operational linkages of the previous risk factors and therapeutic possibilities. For the first time, many facts and observations made sense. The model showed the logic of various strategies in combatting the disease, too. One could deprive the mosquito of its habitat by draining or poisoning swamps, or one might try to block maturation of the parasite by providing quinine (extracted from cinchona bark) to the population at risk. Quarantine even became a logical possibility.

The diagrams illustrate the contemporary model of malaria. The first diagram shows the causal pattern of the disease. Each factor is denoted by a box and influences directly the others to which it connects. As the model was worked out, it yielded new

NINETEENTH-CENTURY VIEW OF MALARIA

Risk Factors

swamp water	mingling with victims	mosquitos
tropical climate	cold ground	race	night air

Therapeutic Possibilities

move to temperate zone	avoid swamps
chew chinchona bark	sleep surrounded by moving water

In the nineteenth century, physicians and others believed that malaria resulted from a number of causes, or risk factors. A variety of therapeutic possibilities were prescribed.

VIEW OF MALARIA (AFTER ROSS)

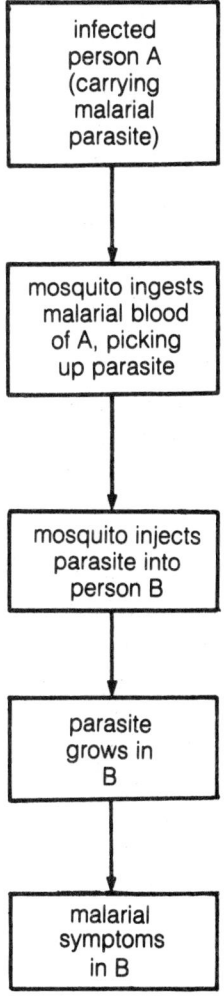

Dr. Ronald Ross discovered the underlying mechanism of how malaria gets transmitted from one person to another.

THERAPEUTIC POSSIBILITIES FOR MALARIA (AFTER ROSS)

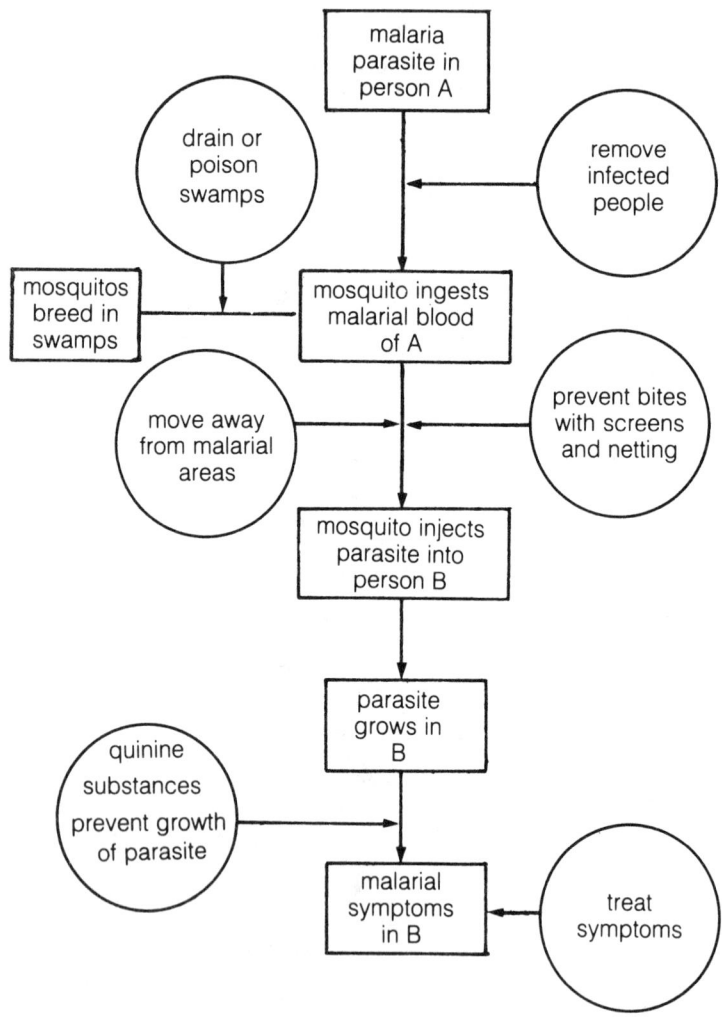

Once Ross worked out the underlying mechanism for malaria, various therapeutic approaches (circles) could be investigated systematically.

predictions and explicit therapeutic recommendations, shown within circles in the second diagram. The diagrams are medically useful in summing up the interaction of related factors (what we might call "the topology of causation").

CURRENT VIEWPOINT ON ARTERIOSCLEROSIS

Our contemporary knowledge of arteriosclerotic disease is curiously similar to Burton's understanding of malaria in the 1860s. We contend with a long list of risk factors: high-cholesterol and high-triglyceride diets, sedentary lifestyles, cigarette smoking, obesity, hypertension, stress, and birth control pills.

There is obviously some wisdom underlying the suggestion to mitigate these risk factors, even if the mechanisms are not understood. However, it is critical to decide if there is an underlying mechanism for arteriosclerosis. If so, describing risk factors rather than the mechanism will miss the point. In the practical effort to cure malaria, the nocturnal, parasite-bearing mosquito struck at the essence of the disease and was worth whole encyclopedias of statistical inferences concerning variables such as ground temperature or width of the protective zone of moving water.

In the field of arteriosclerosis, most workers have chosen the risk-factor approach. This was graphically demonstrated to us by a professor of nutrition at a leading university who is an expert on vitamins and vitamin therapy. His opinions on arteriosclerosis and diet helped to illuminate the fundamental obstacles facing the homocysteine theory or any other unitary theory.

It is probably less useful to talk about the cause of arteriosclerosis than about risk factors. I don't think it is going to be due to one cause. The original workers were probably right when they looked at fats and fatty acids. To this day high serum triglyceride is the best predictor of coronary problems. Also, high sucrose [refined sugar] intake, particularly where it represents 50 percent or more of the daily intake of calories, as in places in Latin America, can be very important. Exercise too is enormously helpful in preventing coronaries. It is hard to say how, but the mobilization of fat and the hormonal balance is quite different in people who exercise than people who don't. We also tend to look only at the end point where a vessel has blown up or blocked off. But this is more of a chronic problem. Some animals on a nutritionally perfect diet get atheromas and others on high risk regimens are resistant. This is complicated.

We asked specifically about vitamin B_6.

I don't think that B_6 will turn out to be of major significance. Low B_6 in coronary patients is correlative, not the cause. Arteriosclerosis can be induced in all kinds of ways. There's lots of B_6 in our diet. If you cook liver the right way, by sautéeing it, you'll have plenty of B_6. A clear example where the B_6 hypothesis breaks down is with women on the Pill. There, it is well known that B_6 levels are reduced. We now have women who have been on the Pill for 20 years who don't have a higher incidence of coronaries.

I think that the B_6 daily requirement should be raised, just as I think the vitamin C requirement of 45 mg daily is too low. But at worst, we have marginal B_6 intake, not deficiencies.

What about homocysteine?

I've heard the homocysteine story. Methionine is the starting point of many important metabolic reactions. But the problem is that as scientists we tend to look at only one thing at a time. With arteriosclerosis, there is still a lot that has to be done, even though so much money has already been spent. Arteriosclerosis is a multi-factor disease. And so that's the way it should be studied. I think an animal model should be developed which looked at many factors together. Design a high-fat diet, with low exercise, and high stress, and perform experiments on rats (primates would be too expensive), which don't get coronaries although you can find fibrous plaque and yellow streaks. I'd like to see them keel over.

The conversation took place a month before publication of the first epidemiological studies showing that oral contraceptive use (which the professor knew leads to vitamin B$_6$ deficiency) *was* associated with a high incidence of coronaries. But the studies of women using the contraceptive pill merely added a new fact. The main difference between the approach in this book and that of the professor is not a specific fact or set of facts but a point of view. When we look at the data from the perspective of the homocysteine theory, we see the same facts but interpret them differently. Since vitamin B$_6$ is in many foods, the professor did not think that people could be deficient (he sat on a Food and Drug Administration committee concerned with the toxicity of vitamin B$_6$). But when the theory makes us look more closely at the data in Chapter 7, we will see that many people suffer insufficient vitamin B$_6$ intake. We therefore attribute more significance than the professor does to the fact that coronary patients are particularly vitamin B$_6$ deficient. Since he hasn't selected any underlying mechanism for arteriosclerosis, the data and claimed observations all receive equal weight. Different facts are sorted into individual risk-factor pigeonholes, but are not assessed in a synthetic way. We think this is unprofitable. We hold quite the opposite position. Wherever possible, arteriosclerosis must be looked at one potential cause at a time, so that primary and secondary effects can be identified.

When all is said, could there be any proof of a particular underlying mechanism for arteriosclerosis which would satisfy the professor by explaining his mountain of facts (some of which are not true)? We think not. At best, he would add another risk to his ever growing list.

And this is endemic in the field. When the Nutrition Committee of the American Heart Association wrote a rebuttal to George Mann's article in the *New England Journal of Medicine,* they concluded: "Since coronary heart disease risk is multifactorial, it may be difficult to alter only one variable (plasma cholesterol and cholesterol, low-density lipoprotein), ignore others such as smoking and hypertension, and expect significant alteration of the dependent variable, coronary heart disease. Physicians often must make decisions in the absence of absolutely conclusive scientific proof. A reasoned resolution of the controversy is not currently possible."

Even when we talked to an open-minded but skeptical epidemiologist about the possibility of a single underlying mechanism, he replied, "It's possible, but we've been burnt before." He was, of course, referring to cholesterol.

The list of risk factors continues to grow. Dr. G. J. Meyers has carried medicine by risk factor to the extreme (Groom 1967):

THUMBNAIL SKETCH OF THE MAN LEAST LIKELY TO HAVE CORONARY HEART DISEASE

An effeminate municipal worker or embalmer,
Completely lacking in physical and mental alertness
and without drive, ambition or competitive
spirit who has never attempted to meet a
deadline of any kind.
A man with poor appetite, subsisting on fruit and
vegetables laced with corn and whale oils,
Detesting tobacco,
Spurning ownership of radio, TV, or motorcar,
With full head of hair and
Scrawny and unathletic in appearance
Yet constantly straining his puny muscles by
exercise;
Low in income, blood sugar, uric acid,
cholesterol and blood pressure,
Who has been taking nicotinic acid, pyridoxine and
long term anticoagulant therapy
Ever since his prophylactic castration.

For arteriosclerosis, the present generally accepted view strongly resembles the early nineteenth-century view of malaria. It is vague and seemingly multicausal. Physicians see that arteriosclerosis is complex and they are skeptical of simplifica-

CURRENT VIEW OF ARTERIOSCLEROSIS (MULTIPLE CAUSES)

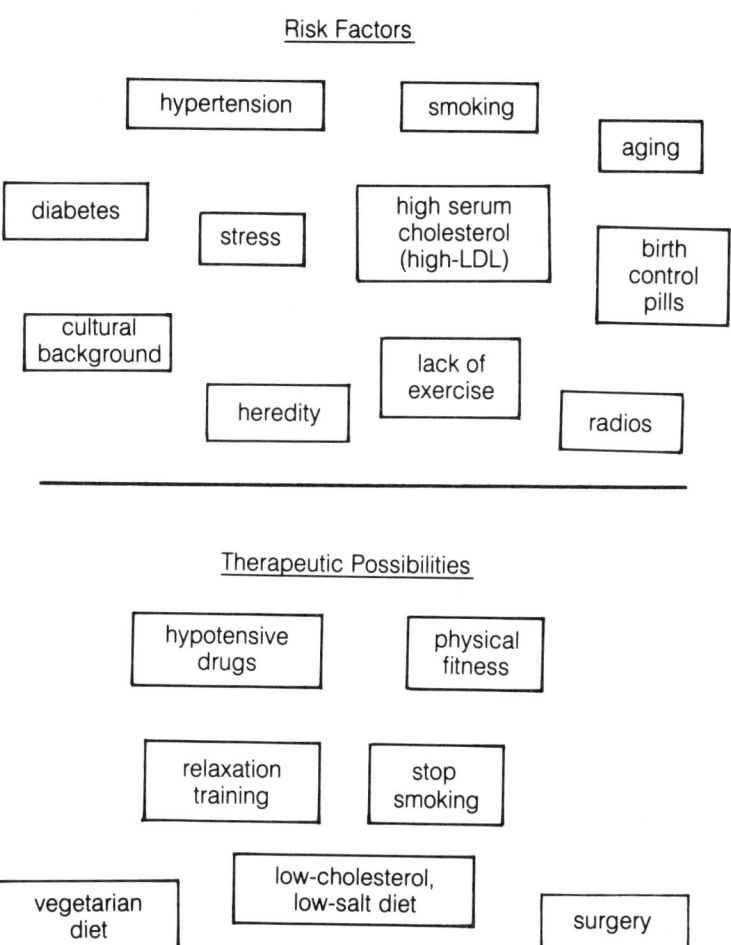

As with the 19th-century view of malaria, arteriosclerosis has many risk factors associated with it. Epidemiologists have even shown that societies with a high number of radios per capita tend to have a high incidence of arteriosclerosis. Below are some therapeutic strategies.

VIEW OF ARTERIOSCLEROSIS USING HOMOCYSTEINE THEORY

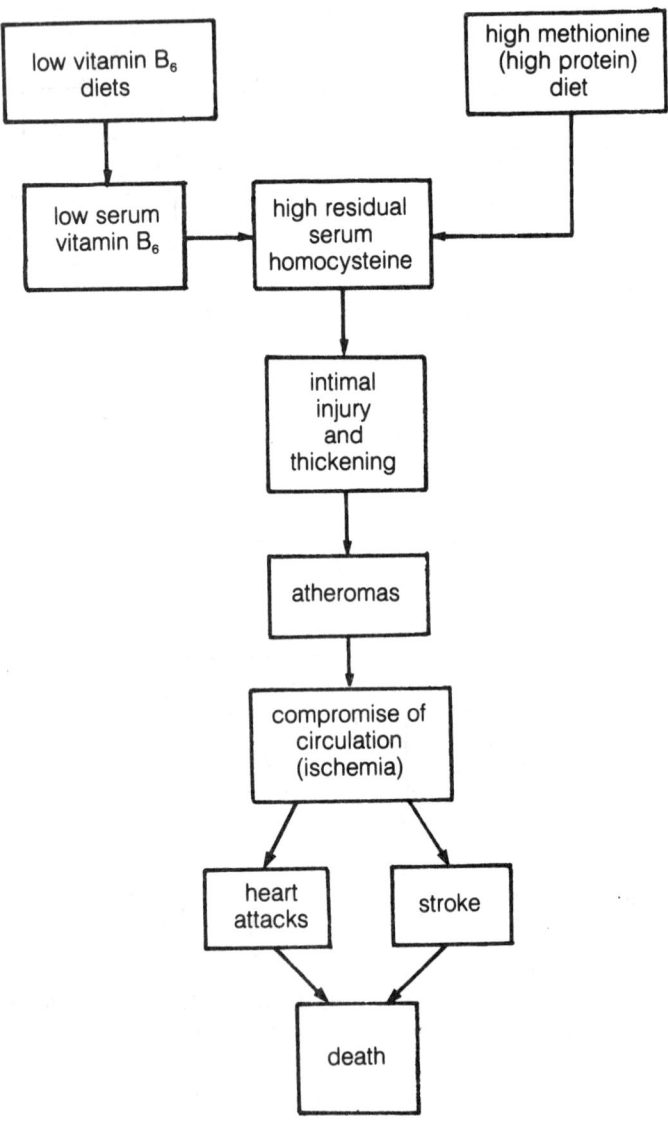

The mechanism underlying the homocysteine theory.

THERAPEUTIC POSSIBILITIES USING THE HOMOCYSTEINE THEORY

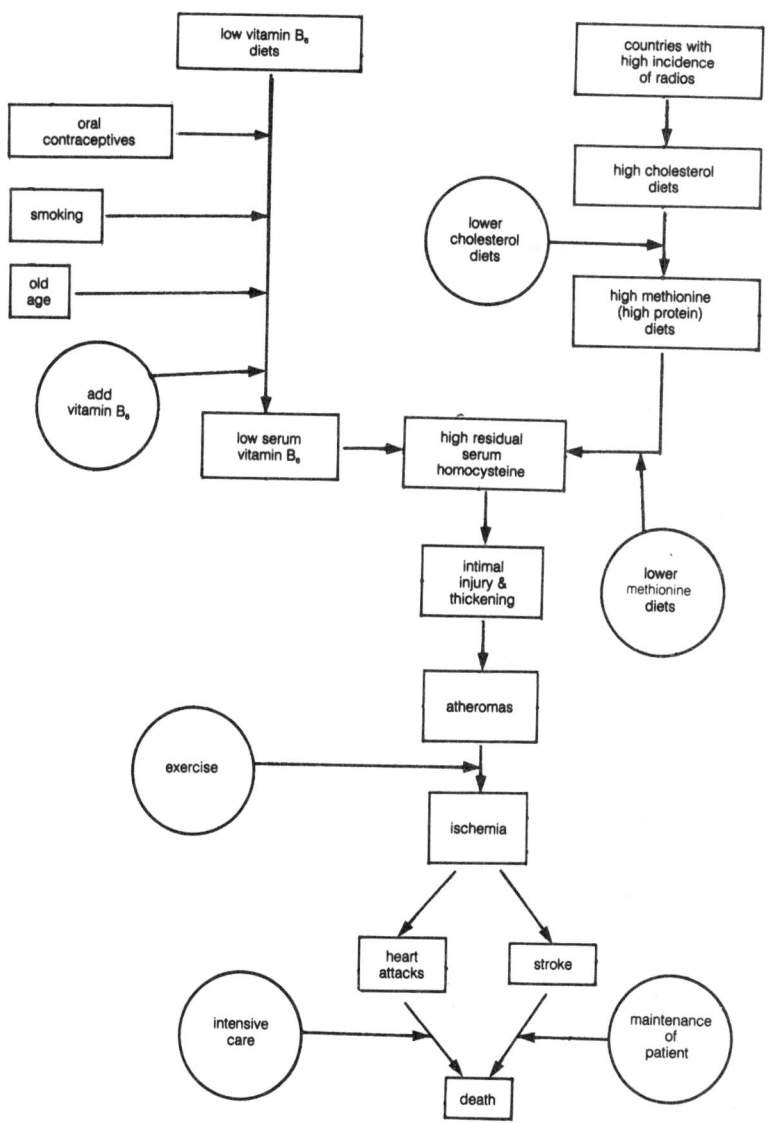

Therapeutic strategies can be viewed within the framework of the homocysteine theory.

tion. The risk factors and therapeutic possibilities are summarized in the diagram.

The homocysteine theory of arteriosclerosis suggests an underlying mechanism and, then, connects the risk factors and therapies. Diets high in protein and low in vitamin B_6 lead to high levels of homocysteine in the blood, which leads to arterial damage and clinical consequences. Once we establish the framework, we can then assess the risk factors and see which are critical.

The block diagrams show that it is more useful to view the development of arteriosclerosis as a consequence of an interconnected mechanism rather than a single cause. If there is only a single cause, it suggests that one need not be concerned with influences exerted elsewhere in the process. What is important is to discover the limiting steps in the process of the disease. It is perhaps better to talk of distant and near effects, depending on how close they are to the crucial steps. Thus, ruling out cholesterol as a cause is not especially useful except as it forces a change in point of view. But if high methionine intake and low vitamin B_6 intake are the conditions that more directly produce the disease in human populations, then they are the limiting steps—steps where control will be most effective. Dietary cholesterol may cause the disease under unusual conditions in the laboratory, but the evidence suggests that it has marginal effects in human populations.

CURRENT RISK FACTORS

We cannot yet explain all known risk factors of arteriosclerosis, but, as we will now elaborate, much fits into the pattern we show in our diagrams.

- *Cholesterol* Our interpretation of pathological findings (of Newburgh, Duff, Friedman, Ross, McCully, and others) is that the initial stages of arteriosclerosis can occur without elevated serum cholesterol. As we showed in Chapter 2, there is little relationship between diet cholesterol and serum cholesterol. Risk of heart disease and intake of dietary cholesterol correlate in epidemiological studies because those foods high in cholesterol are also high in animal protein. In turn, animal protein contains significant amounts of methionine, which the body converts to homocysteine. At some point in later stages of the disease process, there may be an elevation in serum cholesterol. In turn, high serum cholesterol can lead to secondary complications, including increased rates of infiltration of cholesterol into the plaques. It is unclear how unusually high cholesterol diets produce arteriosclerosis in animals, although it is possible that high serum cholesterol may lower vitamin B_6 levels.

• *Age* Heart disease becomes particularly severe in older people and serum vitamin B_6 levels are also considerably reduced. See Chapter 6. Old people, however, continue to consume about the same amounts of methionine-containing foods as they did in earlier life. Many older subjects show overt signs of vitamin B_6 deficiency on their normal diets. Thus older people would therefore be expected to show higher levels of residual homocysteine in the blood, leading to further induction of sclerotic plaques.

• *Hypertension* Some people with normal blood pressure have arteriosclerosis. High blood pressure, however, distorts and mechanically strains arteries. Thus, hypertension may produce injuries in vessel walls, inducing arteriosclerosis. It appears to increase infiltration of cholesterol, making existing plaques worse. Hypertension might be a route to arteriosclerosis in its own right, and so far at least, the homocysteine theory provides no essential or novel insight into the role hypertension plays.

• *Smoking* In Western countries cigarette smoking has been linked to vascular disease. Less well known is the fact that smoking leads to a reduction in serum vitamin B_6. In work done in Canada and Egypt, researchers have shown that cigarette smokers are vitamin B_6 deficient compared to nonsmokers (Kerr et al. 1965; El-Zoghby et al. 1970). Studies by Russian workers suggest that gases in cigarette smoke may be the culprits, for rats exposed to air containing even small amounts of carbon monoxide and nitrogen oxides require increased vitamin B_6 (Nizhegorodov and Markhotski 1971).

Smoking has other effects not related to vitamin B_6. Nicotine constricts arterial vessels, directly affecting blood pressure and vascular diameter. Smoking also affects appetite, which could lead to shifts in diet. It is interesting, however, that the Tukisenta of New Guinea, where heart disease is "rare or absent," are heavy smokers.

- *Oral contraceptives* Oral contraceptive use has been associated with vascular disease. Estrogens lower the level of serum vitamin B_6. In the long run, this can result in a tendency for the blood to have high residual levels of homocysteine and lead to arteriosclerosis. Incidentally, the structure of cholesterol is closely related to that of estrogen (see Chapter 2), and that is why it is possible that high serum cholesterol may lower vitamin B_6 levels. Unfortunately, studies on this question are incomplete.

- *Sex* In most Western countries men are more prone to coronaries and to arteriosclerosis than women. A study by Drs. David Wilcken and V. J. Gupta (1979) of Sydney, Australia, shows that women have significantly lower levels of serum homocysteine than men of the same age. The basis of the difference is not yet clear, but protein intake of men is typically much higher than for women.

- *Alcoholism* Curiously, alcoholics suffering serious liver disease have a lower incidence of severe arteriosclerosis than the normal population or alcoholics without liver disease. Dr. McCully points out there are biochemical consequences of liver disease, including the blocking of the conversion of methionine to homocysteine. The reduced production of homocysteine that follows could lower the incidence of arteriosclerosis.

- *Stress* Scientists in this field are at odds about the importance of stress in vascular hypertension and disease. (A leader of a recent symposium proposed that the more expert one was in stress research the less certain one felt that stress was a significant risk factor.) If we assume that during World War II the people of Nazi-occupied Holland and Norway and block-aded Finland were under equal or greater stress than they were before the war, then the steep drop in cardiovascular disease during the war cannot easily be explained by a stress hypothesis. Stress, especially of the acute sort experienced during an emotional outburst, strongly affects the heart rate and could increase demand for blood by the heart muscle. Existing arteriosclerosis could make the demand impossible to fulfill, resulting in a heart attack. Thus stress may sharpen the impact of arteriosclerosis but there is little agreement that it *causes* vascular lesions.

- *Exercise* Recent evidence from both Israel and the United States shows that lack of exercise strongly correlates with heart disease. How and why exercise helps is unclear. It has been argued by Dr. George Mann and other observers that African populations, such as the Masai, who have low rates of coronaries, don't necessarily have less severely sclerotic arteries. They argue that the arteries enlarge with sufficient exercise, making complete block more difficult. (There are, of course, other societies with relatively little arteriosclerosis whose members tend to be physically active.)

We are not convinced that exercise is the critical factor in preventing coronary disease. Even regular marathon running is not sufficient to free people of arteriosclerosis. Dr. T. Noakes and colleagues in South Africa found severe arteriosclerosis in several marathon runners who had died in accidents or while running. And tennis professional Arthur Ashe, who was superbly conditioned from daily practice, had a heart attack at the age of 35 and underwent triple bypass coronary artery surgery. (One might argue that if he had not exercised, Ashe's symptoms could have occurred even earlier or been more severe, but it is hard to know.)

For the general population, regular, sustained moderate exercise seems to provide beneficial effect. But we cannot rule out the proposition that healthy people tend to exercise, rather than that exercise tends to make people healthy.

In an interesting development, Dr. James Leklem of

Oregon State University recently obtained preliminary evidence showing that exercise increases serum vitamin B_6 levels.

- *Diabetes* There is a strong link between coronary heart disease and diabetes. Drs. R. G. Wilson and R. E. Davis (1977) at the Royal Perth Hospital and the University of Western Australia showed that the average serum vitamin B_6 level is about 35 percent lower in diabetics than in normal people. Could it be that diabetics suffer general vitamin deficiency? No. The Australians measured the level of another B vitamin, folate, and found that there is little difference in amounts between normal people and diabetics. So it appears that the vitamin B_6 deficiency observed in diabetics does not originate in a general vitamin deficiency. The vitamin B_6 deficiency could thus lead to high levels of serum homocysteine, accounting for the greater incidence of arteriosclerosis observed in diabetics.

- *Animal versus vegetable protein* A number of epidemiological studies show that vegetarians have a lower incidence of coronary heart disease than meat-eaters. The usual explanation is that vegetarians have lower cholesterol intake. But they also have a lower intake of methionine. On the average, vegetable protein has proportionately less methionine than animal protein (see table in Chapter 7). In addition, the ratio of vitamin B_6 to methionine is almost uniformly higher in vegetable products than in animal products. Thus, vegetarians have two dietary advantages: less methionine in their protein and a greater proportion of vitamin B_6 per milligram of methionine ingested. We expect that they will therefore have lower residual levels of homocysteine in their blood than meat eaters.

- *Azaribine* The drug Azaribine has been used for treating psoriasis. In 1977, however, the Food and Drug Administration prohibited its use after finding that users had increased incidence of thromboembolism. Five of 13 psoriatic patients on a regimen of Azaribine developed both homocystinuria and homocystinemia (Shupack et al. 1977). None of 16 psoriatic controls, who never used Azaribine, developed homo-cystinuria or any vascular problem. This drug is obviously a rather exotic risk, but it is interesting that homocysteine again appears to be the link between the risk factor and the vascular problem.

SKEPTICISM AND REJECTION

There are always new medical "cures" that burst on the scene like a firework, then rapidly fade out. It is prudent to be skeptical and not subscribe blindly to each supposed cure. As Hippocrates said, "One must attend in medical practice not primarily to plausible theories, but to experience combined with reason." At the present time, the homocysteine theory is a plausible theory. The medical profession has learned the wisdom of restraint and is intrinsically conservative. From the physician's viewpoint, arteriosclerosis has many signs and many contradictions. The physician has the responsibility of deciding the best therapy for each patient, and "best" has to satisfy several conditions. The therapy must be accepted by the medical community; it must be accepted by the patient; and it must fall within certain monetary limits. Today, doctors and patients agree that the combination of low-fat diets, moderate exercise, stopping of smoking, good nutrition (variously de-fined), constitute the best therapy.

We would suggest, however, that experience combined with reason has *not* shown that therapy by eliminating risk factors has produced clearly beneficial results. Caution is not the same as immediate rejection and the homocysteine theory deserves to be considered. Arteriosclerosis has not been conquered and the prevailing therapeutic assumptions are simply not good enough. The inability to go beyond risk factors has blocked a deeper understanding of arteriosclerosis.

CHAPTER 6

Establishing a Recommended Daily Allowance for Vitamin B$_6$

O$_{UR}$ FUNDAMENTAL PREMISE is that homocysteine is the pivotal molecule in the mechanism underlying arteriosclerosis. If we are correct, then the reasonable strategy in preventing the disease is to keep the concentration of serum homocysteine as low as possible. Since vitamin B$_6$ is required to metabolize the amino acid, it is obviously important to know how much vitamin B$_6$ is needed to keep the blood relatively clear of residual homocysteine. Practically, we must determine what intake of vitamin B$_6$ is sufficient to give us a safe daily allowance—a subject as close to us as the side of a box of breakfast cereal. But, surprising as it may seem, no one has yet performed the necessary explicit experiments.

Recommended dietary allowances (RDAs) of various vitamins are suggested by the Food and Nutrition Board of the National Academy of Sciences–National Research Council (NAS–NRC), which is "a nongovernmental U.S. organization of scientists established by an act of Congress to serve as an official advisor to the government upon request in all matters of science and technology." The RDAs of the Food and Nutrition Board are "value judgments based on the existing knowledge of nutritional science . . . subject to revision as new knowledge becomes available." The Board has established an RDA for vitamin B$_6$ at 2.2 mg per day for all males above age 18, and 2.0 mg per day for all females above age 18 with the exception of pregnant and lactating women (for these groups, the RDA is respectively 2.6 mg and 2.5 mg a day). "The RDAs are those that, in the opinion of the Food and Nutrition Board, will maintain good nutrition in practically all healthy persons in the United States. . . . The allowances are designed to afford a margin sufficiently above average physiological requirements to cover variations among practically all individuals in the general population. The allowances provide a buffer against increased needs during stresses and permit full realization of growth and productive potential."

The RDA for vitamin B_6 was established without regard for possible cardiovascular effects of the vitamin. Further, no measures were made of homocysteine levels in the serum. We will show that the assumptions and methods used to establish the present official RDA for vitamin B_6 are of dubious value and certainly do not provide a margin of safety to cover the general population. We will then discuss why a higher RDA is called for.

A HYPOTHETICAL METHOD FOR ASSESSING ADEQUATE VITAMIN B_6 INTAKE

Vitamin B_6 is necessary for metabolizing not only homocysteine, but about 40 other compounds as well. Let us consider how we would determine what an adequate human daily vitamin B_6 intake would be. (We will assume we have an unlimited amount of time and resources to make this determination.) We would want to know how much vitamin B_6 is sufficient for rapid removal of homocysteine and to give optimal function of all the enzymes that depend on the vitamin. For our determination, we would examine many putatively healthy people and measure the serum levels of the 40 compounds produced by chemical reactions requiring vitamin B_6. We would then give these people experimental diets that contained varying quantities of vitamin B_6, ranging from very little to much more than anyone could eat in natural foods.

From the results of preliminary studies already conducted, we know that with very low vitamin B_6 intake, the blood levels of some compounds, dependent on vitamin B_6 (such as homocysteine), are in too high a concentration and others (serotonin is one) are too low. This has toxic effects and produces overt symptoms of vitamin B_6 deficiency.

As vitamin B_6 intake is increased, these compounds move from extreme levels toward "normal." With sufficient vitamin B_6 intake, there is a safe range with no significant changes in the concentrations of the various compounds. In this range any excess intake of the vitamin is either stored or excreted. If the intake were increased still further, one would expect the concentrations of various compounds to reach abnormal levels. At still higher vitamin B_6 intake, toxic effects might occur.

Given the diversity of the population, different individuals need different dietary amounts of vitamin B_6 to obtain the "normal" blood concentrations of the 40 vitamin B_6-dependent compounds. If we did extensive enough tests, we could find that at low levels of vitamin B_6 intake some people might have abnormal levels of some compounds, while other people could have abnormal levels of a different group of the 40 compounds. Our tests of blood levels could even detect people who were vitamin B_6 deficient on their usual diet. It would be appropriate to group these individuals and study their genetic background for enzyme deficiencies. The tests would also reveal how other components of the diet, particularly protein, affect the optimal dose of vitamin B_6. One could then determine how vitamin B_6 requirements vary with people under different conditions: women on the contraceptive pill, old people, young people, males/females, people with various illnesses.

Such comprehensive tests have not been carried out. With even limited imagination, researchers could make the task almost unending. They could probe for a relation between intake of vitamin B_6 and hundreds of variables. But such studies would serve no pressing need. As far as we know, only the relation between vitamin B_6 and homocysteine level is associated with a serious potential danger. Present knowledge of this particular relation is quite limited and even a modest amount of work in this area would yield important new information. The broader question of what constitutes a generally adequate level of vitamin B$_6$ with respect to all 40 compounds is also still very sparsely answered.

ACTUAL TESTS USED TO DETERMINE RDA OF VITAMIN B$_6$ INTAKE

The first serious tests conducted to determine sufficient levels of vitamin B$_6$ intake were carried out years before the homocysteine theory had been proposed. The strategy in the experiments was to reduce intake of vitamin B$_6$ in human subjects until there were overt clinical signs of deficiency. Subjects were then given controlled daily doses of vitamin B$_6$ until all signs of deficiency disappeared. Dr. Richard Vilter and his colleagues at the University of Cincinnati Medical College used this approach in a study published in 1953. These researchers used a vitamin B$_6$ antagonist, desoxypyridoxine, a compound that replaces vitamin B$_6$ but does not have any enzyme activity. The patients took desoxypyridoxine daily until they developed clinical deficiencies. Different patients developed different deficiencies, which the Vilter team carefully described.

The most common first sign of deficiency (in 25 of the 50 volunteer patients, who were stoic individuals, as we will see) was "seborrheic dermatitis," with the skin becoming red and rough. There were accompanying sensations of itching and burning and clearly visible greasy scales. The dermatitis usually began around the mouth and on the chin. Frequently, it then spread over the entire face, behind the ears, onto the scalp, down the neck, over the shoulders, in the perineal region (the pelvic floor), and over the buttocks.

In five patients the first sign of deficiency was "glossitis," where the tongue felt as if it had been scalded by hot coffee. Within 24 hours, the papillae (the elevations on the surface of the tongue) reddened at the tip of the tongue. Later the tongue swelled sufficiently to smooth out the rodlike structure of the papillae into red dots.

In one patient the first sign of deficiency was severe sensory neuritis (two others also eventually developed this symptom).

The neuritis started as a tingling and numbness in the hands and feet. Then within four to five days the patients' hands, arms, legs, and feet became hypersensitive to pinprick and the patients developed other neurological symptoms. At night the patients felt sensations of burning and electric shocks, particularly in their feet. These sensations forced them to kick off the bed covers. Most patients also developed anorexia, drowsiness, and nausea in the deficiency state.

Once taken off desoxypyridoxine and given 5 to 200 mg of pyridoxine daily, most patients lost their clinical symptoms within a week. But even after pyridoxine treatment eliminated all physical signs, patients with vitamin B_6-deficiency-neuritis continued to experience "hot foot" or "electric foot." American prisoners of war in the Pacific during World War II similarly complained of the same symptom after long periods of insufficient diets. Gradually, over a period of several months, the symptoms subsided.

The researchers also conducted chemical tests for vitamin B_6 deficiency. To explore various chemical reactions controlled by vitamin B_6, they used a "tryptophan load" test. Normally, the body uses the amino acid tryptophan to produce a variety of other compounds, including serotonin. As we mentioned earlier, during vitamin B_6 deficiency the body produces less serotonin. Another tryptophan product is xanthurenic acid. It was known that excess amounts of this acid appear in the urine of rats if they are fed a vitamin B_6-deficient diet (Lepkovsky et al. 1943). On the face of it, it is peculiar that production of xanthurenic acid increases during vitamin B_6 deficiency since xanthurenic acid is also dependent on a chemical step that requires the presence of vitamin B_6 as a co-enzyme. However, biochemists have determined that the enzyme which produces xanthurenic acid binds the vitamin B_6 more tightly than other vitamin B_6 dependent enzymes. Thus it remains effective during vitamin B_6 deficiency and xanthurenic acid is generated preferentially. The various pathways for tryptophan metabolism and the particular steps which require vitamin B_6 are shown in the diagram.

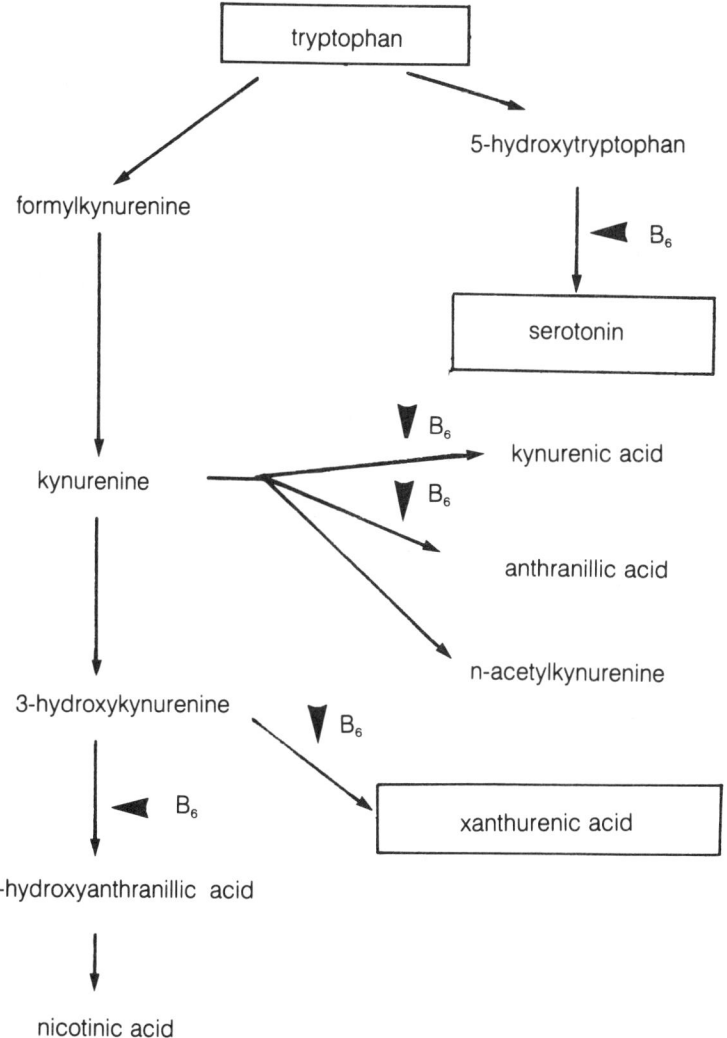

This biochemical chart shows how tryptophan is metabolized to a variety of compounds including serotonin and xanthurenic acid. The steps requiring vitamin B₆ are marked with arrowheads. During vitamin B₆ deficiency more xanthurenic acid is produced and less serotonin is produced.

Vilter's group found that 30 of 34 patients tested excreted large amounts of xanthurenic acid under a desoxypyridoxine (and hence vitamin B_6 deficiency) regimen. Since most researchers generally regarded excessive xanthurenic acid excretion as a sign of vitamin B_6 deficiency, Vilter's group wanted to determine if it was in fact a sensitive and early test. Twenty of the 34 patients studied for excess xanthurenic acid production developed clinical signs of deficiency. Sixteen developed these signs either concurrently or after an increase of xanthurenic acid production. Four patients developed signs of deficiency before any increase of xanthurenic acid excretion. Thus, excess xanthurenic acid excretion was a fairly reliable—but not infallible—test of vitamin B_6 deficiency as determined by clinical signs. This finding was in keeping with earlier studies on animals.

Samuel Lepkovsky, who had shown that vitamin B_6-deficient rats produced xanthurenic acid, also found that the rats developed dermatitis and died quite rapidly. He suggested that perhaps the tryptophan in the diet caused both dermatitis and early death in pyridoxine-deficient rats. However, Dr. Leopold Cerecedo and colleagues at Fordham University in 1950 showed on the contrary that early onset of dermatitis and death were caused not by tryptophan but by certain other amino acids, which contain sulfur. Appropriately enough in light of the subject of this book, the toxic amino acids were methionine and homocystine. Rats deficient in vitamin B_6 and fed either methionine or homocystine rapidly developed dermatitis and died. But other rats deficient in vitamin B_6 and fed tryptophan lived. Nonetheless, when animals consume protein, ingestion of tryptophan parallels ingestion of methionine so xanthurenic acid production may be an indirect indication of dangerous vitamin B_6 deficiency.

The clinical signs Vilter's group found were assumed to be the only serious manifestations of vitamin B_6 deficiency in humans. But they did not look at other conditions, including the one we would now consider critical: signs of arteriosclerosis.

Vilter concluded that "since 5 mg pyridoxine is sufficient to heal lesions of vitamin B_6 deficiency induced by 200 mg of desoxypyridoxine in a patient whose diet contains approximately ½ mg pyridoxine, one may deduce that more than ½ mg and less than 5 mg will meet requirements of adult human beings very satisfactorily." (Strictly speaking, he should have said "less than 5½ mg" instead of less than 5 mg.)

Vilter's studies resulted in defining a level of vitamin B_6 required to eliminate some overt deficiencies. But the level could be less than sufficient to meet the standards of the RDA to give a margin of safety to *all* individuals. There were several unstated assumptions in the experiment. For instance, desoxypyridoxine may have produced other effects, in addition to blocking the action of vitamin B_6. Also, the deficiencies found were assumed to be the only ill-effects caused by vitamin B_6 deficiency. Dr. Vilter and his colleagues could not *a priori* exclude other deficiencies. In addition, they looked only at short-term effects of deficiencies. (Arteriosclerosis, of course, is slow to develop.) Also, we must be assured that the subjects of this test were truly representative of the general population. Reasonably, a daily dose of approximately 5 mg gives a tentative first estimate for a recommended daily allowance, although there is no reason to expect all *other* deficiencies to disappear just when the deficiency being monitored disappears.

The NAS–NRC Food and Nutrition Board's ad hoc Committee on Vitamin B_6 Requirements wanted a more precise value for the recommended daily allowance for vitamin B_6. They supervised a study by Dr. Eugene Baker and his colleagues at the U.S. Army Medical Research and Nutrition Laboratory of Fitzsimmons General Hospital in Denver. The experiment was designed using the assumption that excretion of abnormal quantities of xanthurenic acid after tryptophan load was a sufficient indicator of vitamin B_6 deficiency, an assumption for which Vilter had already found counterexamples in human tests and Cerecedo had questioned in animal tests.

In a report published in 1964 Baker and colleagues described a study involving eight healthy young male adults (they started with 11 subjects but three dropped out halfway through the 14-

week study). The subjects were divided into two groups. All were given a liquid diet. One group ate 100 grams of protein per day and the other group ate 30 grams of protein per day. Initially, they were all given 4 mg of pyridoxine each day for one week. Then they were given no daily pyridoxine until 80 percent of the subjects excreted a minimum of 200 mg a day of xanthurenic acid in response to a tryptophan load. (Before deficiency, the subjects excreted an average of approximately 20 mg per day of xanthurenic acid.) The high protein group took only three weeks to reach the vitamin B_6 deficiency criterion of 200 mg per day of xanthurenic acid. But it took six weeks for the low-protein diet group deprived of vitamin B_6 to reach criterion deficiency. Each group was then given just enough vitamin B_6 so that individuals excreted a normal concentration of xanthurenic acid. It was found that the high protein group needed slightly more than 1.5 mg pyridoxine per day and the low protein group needed about 1.25 mg pyridoxine per day. (The researchers also found that adding extra methionine in the diet led to an abrupt increase in excretion of xanthurenic acid.) The study concluded with the suggestion that people on high-protein diets (100 gm per day) should have approximately 1.75 to 2 mg of vitamin B_6 per day and those on a low-protein diet should have 1.25 to 1.5 mg vitamin B_6 per day.

Baker's study showed two important facts rather well. First, *high-protein diets aggravate a vitamin B_6 deficiency* and second, *increasing vitamin B_6 intake will compensate for increased quantities of dietary protein.* Baker's group was careful not to overstate the generality of their findings: "It must be emphasized that the requirements for vitamin B_6 established herein pertain only to the diet and conditions described in the study. The vitamin B_6 requirement of persons existing on a normal dietary intake may be different from that given here due to many variables."

The Baker and Vilter studies are helpful, but they are preliminary. The Baker study used only eight subjects, a very small number. All were male and young. Vilter's subjects were volunteer patients who were in the hospital because of various illnesses.

Neither study investigated whether 2 mg per day of vitamin B₆ prevents the appearance of homocysteine in the blood. Neither study determined the variability of vitamin B₆ requirements in the population. Vilter's study showed different people develop different vitamin B₆ deficiencies after different amounts of time. It seems likely also that different people require different levels of pyridoxine intake to prevent deficiencies from developing.

To generalize from these studies done on small, not particularly representative groups, is wrong-headed. Yet on the basis of these studies (and several unpublished and therefore unscrutinizable works), the NAS–NRC recommended 2 to 2.2 mg per day of vitamin B₆ for all non-pregnant non-lactating adult Americans. One wonders why an additional margin wasn't added for safety. We will discuss this question further in the next chapter, but there is a short practical answer. It is barely possible for the normal American diet to contain 2 to 2.2 mg per day of vitamin B₆. A higher RDA would almost certainly require the awkward step of recommending vitamin B₆ supplements.

A further curiosity about the RDA for vitamin B₆ were reports, referred to by NAS–NRC, of signs of deficiency in diets consisting of approximately 2 mg per day of vitamin B₆. Dr. R.S. Harding and his colleagues (from the same research laboratory as Baker) reported in 1959 that after 24 days volunteers fed a daily diet of Army C-rations containing 1.93 mg of pyridoxine showed an increase in xanthurenic acid excretion after a tryptophan load test three times that of other volunteers who had either daily pyridoxine intake of 2.76 mg in their C-rations or were fed a different diet containing 4.28 mg per day of vitamin B₆.

More recently, Professor Judy Driskell (1976) and her colleagues at the Department of Food and Nutrition of Florida State University at Tallahassee studied normal college students eating their own normal diets. They then measured the activity of an enzyme dependent on vitamin B_6. In some students extra vitamin B_6 increased the activity of this enzyme, whereas in other students extra vitamin B_6 had no effect on the activity of the enzyme. The first group thus appeared to be deficient in vitamin B_6 relative to the second group. Interestingly, some students whose daily intake of vitamin B_6 was greater than 2.4 mg could still raise the activity of the enzyme by increasing their intake of vitamin B_6. The investigators concluded that among the subjects there were "large differences in individual vitamin B_6 requirements. Many of the subjects exhibited evidence of subclinical vitamin B_6 deficiencies at various reported intakes of the vitamin."

Thus, there seems to be nothing sacred about the 2 to 2.2 mg per day vitamin B_6 recommendation. It is a Procrustean solution to the arbitrary problem of coming up with numbers for daily requirements of vitamin B_6 for non-pregnant, non-lactating adults.

Other scientists who have studied the issue have also questioned the adequacy of the RDA for vitamin B_6. In 1964 at an international symposium to celebrate the thirtieth anniversary of the discovery of vitamin B_6 (chaired by its discoverer, Paul Gyorgy), Henry Borsook of the California Institute of Technology reviewed the literature on recommended daily allowance and suggested that the range should be 2.5 to 7 mg daily. At the same conference W.H. Sebrell of the Institute of Nutrition Sciences at Columbia University agreed: "The weight of the evidence indicates to me that figures generally used are probably too low to be entirely safe for a large population group subject to a variety of stress situations." In 1971, Dr. Gyorgy himself suggested that the dietary allowance should be increased to 25 mg per day "as a precaution to prevent possible serious pathological conditions."

The studies to determine the RDA of vitamin B_6 remind us of an image once conjured up by A.J. Liebling of "a gigantic, super-modern fish cannery, a hundred floors high, capitalized at eleven billion dollars, and with tens of thousands of workers standing ready at the canning machines, but relying for its raw material on an inadequate number of handline fishermen in leaky rowboats." Liebling was alluding to daily newspapers and news reporters but the same metaphor is appropriate here: The governmental administrative apparatus for deciding the RDA for vitamin B_6 and for disseminating the information is totally out of proportion to the few fishermen procuring the data. The NAS–NRC publishes a scholarly book complete with bibliography with recommended daily allowances for various vitamins. That book influences people in an immediate way. Your morning corn flakes have been fortified with a certain amount of vitamin B_6 because of the recommendations in that book. Vitamin pills for adults and children contain particular amounts of vitamin B_6 because of the recommendations that come out of that book. Yet the evidence is flimsy and full of holes.

AGE AND VITAMIN B_6

It is not our intent to carp. We criticize the official RDA for vitamin B_6 not only on academic grounds, but also because serious evidence shows that the RDA is not high enough to take into account the variations of individual needs within the population. As was shown in the Florida State study, 2 to 2.2 mg daily is not even sufficient vitamin B_6 intake for a population of young healthy adults. Even more critical, it is known that the serum level of pyridoxal phosphate, the active form of vitamin B_6, decreases significantly with age. People over the age of 60 have, on the average, half the serum vitamin B_6 as those between ages 30 and 60, and one-fifth the vitamin B_6 of those under one year of age, reported Dr. Arne Hamfelt of Sweden in 1964. When subjected to tryptophan load tests a group of people over age 60 were in the "pathological" range, excreting an average of 15.8 units of xanthurenic acid (Hamfelt considered excretion of no more than 2 units to be within a normal range). By feeding these older people 100 mg of vitamin B_6 daily for a week Hamfelt reduced the xanthurenic acid excreted to an average of 1.6 units. This indicates that vitamin B_6 intake had been too low and that the deficiency was reversible with supplements.

The finding applies not only to older Swedes. A study at Johns Hopkins School of Hygiene and Public Health found similar vitamin B_6 deficiencies among older Americans (Ranke et al. 1960). Fifteen mg of vitamin B_6 daily for three weeks would reduce average xanthurenic acid excretion after tryptophan load to values below that of 25-year-olds. It is not yet known whether lower daily supplements of the vitamin would produce the same effect.

These studies show that old people are sufficiently low in vitamin B_6 that enzyme activities are well below their maximum level, suggesting a real deficiency. Furthermore, Dr. H.M. Hodkinson and Dr. A.N. Exton-Smith (1976), of Northwick Park and University College Hospitals in England, determined factors which best predict mortality within five years in a sample of 852 people over 65 years of age. Both low pyridoxine intake and low serum pyridoxine are significant adverse factors affecting mortality. Other B vitamins—thiamin, riboflavin and nicotinic acid showed no association with mortality.

It is vital to determine the serum homocysteine levels in older people and to gauge amounts of vitamin B_6 needed for their good health. The present RDA for adults makes no distinction between the old and the young. Some private companies making vitamins earmarked for older people are no more careful on this point than NAS–NRC. For instance, Geritol, a vitamin supplement that for years has been targeted for older people has only 0.5 mg vitamin B_6 per dose in its formulation (a scant one-quarter of the RDA), yet the fact that older people need additional vitamin B_6 is amply documented in the published literature.

PREGNANCY AND VITAMIN B_6 RDA

Dr. Robert Cleary and his co-workers in the Department of Obstetrics and Gynecology of Indiana University Medical School determined the level of pyridoxal phosphate in the plasma of non-pregnant women taking no vitamin B_6 supplements versus pregnant women taking daily vitamin B_6 supplements of 2.5 or 10 mg. The pregnant women taking 2.5 mg vitamin B_6 supplements had less serum vitamin B_6 than nonpregnant women who were not taking the vitamin. Even when they increased the dose of vitamin B_6 by a factor of four, the pregnant women taking vitamin B_6 supplements still showed lower blood levels of vitamin B_6 than non-pregnant women. Cleary's group suggested that 2.5 mg daily supplement was not sufficient. The same group suggested that the "current RDA for vitamin B_6 during pregnancy (2.5 mg) is too low and that supplementation of this vitamin in an amount more than 4 mg daily is recommended."

A significant number of pregnant women suffer from morning sickness. Many obstetricians today prescribe vitamin B_6, 25 mg per day, as the favored treatment.

It is also likely that vitamin B_6 is important for fetuses, since fetuses have much higher serum levels of pyridoxal phosphate than adults. Drs. S.F. Contractor and B. Shane of the Charing Cross Hospital Medical School in London measured the level of vitamin B_6 in blood drawn from the umbilical cords of newborns and compared it to the level in the babies' mothers. On the average the mothers had one-fourth the vitamin B_6 of the fetuses and only one-half the level of non-pregnant women or men. Drs. Contractor and Shane concluded that there was a relative vitamin B_6 deficiency during pregnancy. Several other laboratories have confirmed these results.

Lower maternal levels of vitamin B_6 are reflected in lower levels of vitamin B_6 in their infants. The consequences of B_6 deficiency for the newborn could be serious. Also, women with lower levels of vitamin B_6 tend to produce milk that has a lower-than-normal concentration of vitamin B_6. Since we now know that infants and even fetuses can have early indications of arteriosclerosis, it is plausible to think that their mothers were vitamin B_6 deficient. Interestingly, human milk has a lower proportion of methionine than any other animal protein. Thus, an infant drinking cow's milk could be deficient in vitamin B_6

and also take in higher levels of methionine. The homocysteine theory suggests that such an infant would thus be exposed to a potentially toxic condition.

Drs. J. Ejderhamn and A. Hamfelt (1980) of Sundsvall Hospital, Sundsvall, Sweden, compared vitamin B_6 levels in newborn infants of mothers who had or had not taken vitamin B_6 supplements (maximum 6 mg per day). Those infants whose mothers had taken vitamin B_6 supplements had almost twice the serum level of vitamin B_6 compared to infants whose mothers had not taken supplements.

Dr. R. Karlin of the Institut Pasteur, Lyon, France, found that supplementing the diets of lactating women with vitamin B_6 could increase the vitamin B_6 concentration of their milk seven-fold. (On the other hand, a recent study by Dr. M.J. Mellies and colleagues found that nearly tripling daily dietary cholesterol consumption of nursing mothers had no effect on the cholesterol concentration in their milk.)

We have already described how women on the contraceptive pill are vitamin B_6 deficient. Dr. D.P. Rose and colleagues at St. Mary's Hospital Medical School in London found that supplementing the oral contraceptive users' diets with 40 mg daily of pyridoxine for four to eight weeks was sufficient to eliminate the deficiency. (It is not known whether lower daily doses of pyridoxine would be equally effective.)

BLOOD LEVELS OF VITAMIN B_6

So far we have discussed how vitamin B_6 deficiencies can be revealed in a back-handed sort of way: by supplementation of the vitamin. But we have not yet put a reasonable upper boundary on how much vitamin B_6 should be taken. To determine upper limits, Dr. G.E. Boxer and his colleagues measured the blood level of pyridoxal phosphate (the active form of the vitamin) in several subjects. Oral feeding of any form of vitamin B_6 leads to a prompt rise in serum pyridoxal phosphate, but a saturation level is reached on feeding 4 to 7 mg per day of the vitamin. Even a tenfold increase beyond 4 to 7 mg, to 50 to 75 mg a day, does not measurably increase circulating vitamin B_6. This group also found that there is relatively little storage of the excess vitamin B_6 intake because even after large doses, the blood pyridoxal phosphate reaches pretreatment level within a week. Note that daily intake of 4 to 7 mg pyridoxine is significantly higher than the standard of the NAS–NRC.

It seems prudent to take an amount of vitamin B_6 for which some benefit can be suggested. However, to go much beyond the amount which in effect saturates the blood, or is needed to maximize the reactions involving vitamin B_6 does not seem to be incrementally beneficial. Megadoses of vitamin B_6 do not appear to be of additional help. As mentioned earlier, Paul Gyorgy, the discoverer of vitamin B_6, reviewed the need for vitamin B_6. He suggested (1971) that the daily dietary allowance should be increased to "25 mg per day as a precaution to prevent possible serious pathological conditions."

It can be argued that the low levels of vitamin B_6 seen in old people and pregnant women and even coronary patients is normal. It is part of the natural evolutionary process, a normal consequence of individual development and is not pathological. We cannot directly refute such an argument, but neither can such an argument be proved. We would have to make assumptions about what was the normal diet of humans over the millennia in which they evolved. Ideally, one might show that early humans had the same vitamin B_6 "deficiencies" and were not subject to serious effects of arteriosclerosis.

Since we know that arteriosclerosis can be induced with a diet low in vitamin B_6, the conservative course would be to assume that low vitamin B_6 is a condition to be avoided. The recommended daily allowance is based on limited evidence and stands weakly against a background of contradictory findings. Careful experiments and good reasons suggest that average daily intake of vitamin B_6 should be higher than what is officially suggested, somewhere in the range of 5 to 25 mg. Of particular concern are older people, women who are pregnant, lactating, or using the contraceptive pill, and arteriosclerotic patients.

CHAPTER 7

Vitamin B$_6$ and Methionine in Your Diet

IN THIS CHAPTER we can start connecting the homocysteine theory to our own diets. We will look at the dietary distribution of vitamin B$_6$ and of methionine, the amino acid that gives rise to homocysteine. We will show how the common American diet is inadequate from the point of view of the theory. Most of us eat too much methionine and not enough vitamin B$_6$. We will also describe how we can determine the adequacy of our own diets using some simple arithmetic.

MEASUREMENT OF METHIONINE AND VITAMIN B$_6$

It is easy for food chemists to assay the amount of methionine in any particular food, using straightforward chemical tests. The amino acid is stable under various conditions of cooking and processing.

Measurement of a food's vitamin B$_6$ content, on the other hand, is complicated by several factors. Most foods contain vitamin B$_6$ in three closely related forms: pyridoxamine, pyridoxal, and pyridoxine (see diagram). Within the body all three forms are equally well converted into the primary active form of the vitamin, pyridoxal phosphate. Pyridoxamine and pyridoxal, however, are unstable when they are heated. Thus, food containing either of these loses vitamin B$_6$ when cooked. Pyridoxamine and pyridoxal account for most of the vitamin B$_6$ in corn, meats, poultry, fish, milk and milk products, and eggs. The third form, pyridoxine, accounts for more than half of the vitamin B$_6$ in most vegetables, fruits, legumes, nuts, grains,

DIET

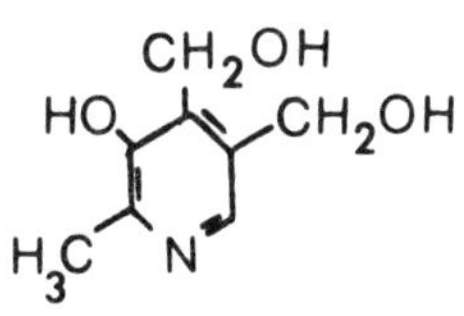

pyridoxine 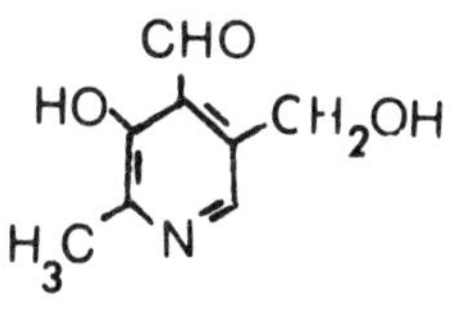 pyridoxal 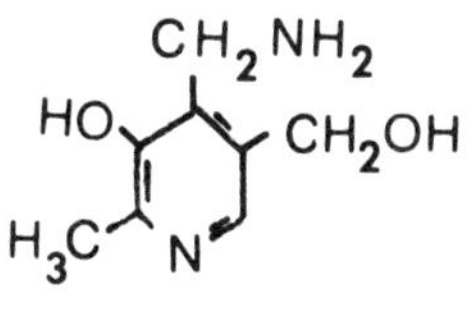 pyridoxamine

BODY

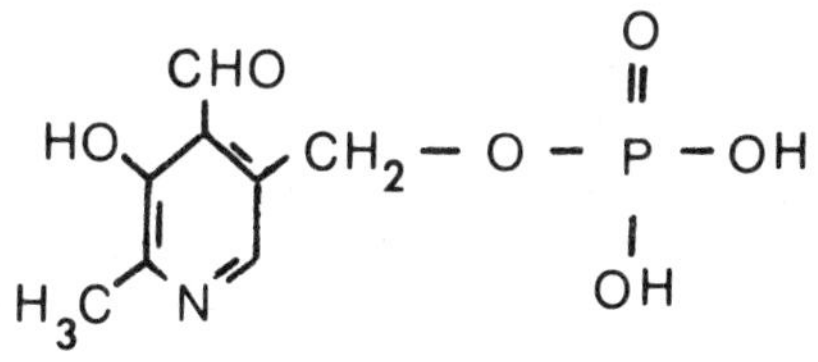

pyridoxal phosphate

top—dietary vitamin B_6 exists in three forms, whose chemical structures are shown here.

bottom—the primary active form of vitamin B_6 in the body is pyridoxal phosphate.

and cereals. Although pyridoxine is much more stable than the other forms when heated, it is lost during refining of food products and when they are exposed to light. And all three forms of dietary vitamin B_6 are water soluble, which means that cooking foods in water will lead to additional loss of vitamin B_6 (unless one also consumes the cooking water). For example, 50 percent of the vitamin B_6 in macaroni dissolves into the cooking water when it is boiled.

HOW VITAMIN B_6 IS MEASURED

Vitamin B_6 can be bound tightly or loosely to other compounds. Thus when determining the B_6 content of foods, what counts is not the absolute amount of vitamin B_6, but the amount that can be made available by the digestive process. The biological and chemical techniques for assaying vitamin B_6 are well known to food chemists.

LOSS OF VITAMIN B_6

Using such tests, it has been found that almost any kind of prepared food has less vitamin B_6 than the raw starting material. Somewhere in the process the food is heated and or immersed in water that is later discarded.

A significant amount of the American diet consists of canned or frozen foods. In 1964, 25.9 billion pounds of food were canned, including 15.5 billion pounds of fruits, vegetables, and juices. That same year 10.7 billion pounds of food (other than seafood) were frozen (Kertesz 1966). In commercial freezing, vegetables are first blanched by brief immersion in boiling water, then quick frozen. In commercial canning, foods are heated and packed hot. After sealing, the cans are heated again to kill microorganisms. The sterilization process can heat the contents to as high as 286°F. Tomato juice after being canned is boiled in water for 15 to 40 minutes. All these techniques, while enhancing the safety of prepared foods, lower their vitamin B_6 content significantly.

AN ACUTE EFFECT

Low vitamin B$_6$ intake generally is a long-term problem and vitamin B$_6$ deficiency does not usually manifest itself immediately. There is, however, one well-documented case of how food canning resulted in a loss of vitamin B$_6$ with serious consequences. In 1950 there was a popular liquid infant milk formula marketed under the name S-M-A liquid concentrate. Wyeth Laboratories, its manufacturer, decided to make several alterations in the formula. To guard against bacterial contamination during manufacture, the new formula was sterilized at a higher temperature than formerly. Within a short period after the new formula was marketed there were reports scattered across the country of infants going into convulsions. All were on a regimen of S-M-A liquid concentrate. Toxicologists could not find a toxic agent in the formula. The product was removed from the market and later it was suggested that the new sterilization process may have reduced vitamin B$_6$ content of the milk. Pyridoxal is the predominant form of vitamin B$_6$ in milk and it is heat-sensitive. Tests determined that the vitamin B$_6$ content had in fact been reduced and the ensuing deficiency accounted for the convulsions. The manufacturer added pyridoxine, the heat-stable form of vitamin B$_6$, to the formula and the product was again marketed with no further reports of convulsions of infants on the formula (Coursin 1955). What is quite surprising about the whole episode, is that while there was a lower vitamin B$_6$ level in the formula associated with convulsions, it wasn't vanishingly small. It was 29 percent of the level in the original formula, which had produced no adverse effects. So the important lesson was that for a susceptible group, improper preparation of food led to a decrease in vitamin B$_6$ and a medical emergency.

In addition to heating, simply storing food at a slightly elevated temperature lowers the vitamin B$_6$ content. The army group at Fitzsimmons Hospital in Denver determined that C-rations stored at 100°F for 20 months lost one-third of their vitamin B$_6$ compared to C-rations stored at 34°F.

Other food handling also leads to losses. In the milling of wheat to white flour 80 to 90 percent of the vitamin B_6 can be lost in the discarded germ and bran. Twenty-one percent of the vitamin B_6 in milk is lost after eight-hour exposure to sunlight.

Additional losses of vitamin B_6 come from final cooking. The loss of vitamin B_6 in cooking meats ranges from 33 to 58 percent (Lushbough et al. 1959). Cooking vegetables leads to a 20 to 30 percent loss (Schroeder 1971). The average loss in the baking of bread is 7 percent (Bunting 1965).

ASSESSING OUR DIETS

We can now calculate not only methionine but also the vitamin B_6 content of foods in our diet. We have included an extensive table (Table 1) of common foods showing, among other things, vitamin B_6 content, methionine content, and size of average food portions. Since the raw food product may contain a misleadingly high amount of vitamin B_6 compared to its cooked version, we have included in a separate table (Table 2) average losses of vitamin B_6 as a result of freezing, canning, and final cooking.

It is appropriate to remember that Eskimos leading traditional lives have little arteriosclerosis despite huge intakes of both cholesterol and animal protein. We suggest that they are protected from vascular disease because the vitamin B_6 content of their food is not compromised by cooking or processing. They eat fresh, raw food.

Table 1

VITAMIN B₆, METHIONINE, PROTEIN— CONTENT AND H-VALUE OF FOODS

(from Orr 1969; Church and Church 1975; Geigy 1970; USDA 1978; Kirschmann1975)

Food	mg B₆ /100 gms	mg methionine / 100 gms	gm protein /100 gm	H-value ratio of B₆ to methionine ×1000	standard portion
almonds	.10	260	18.6	.38	1 cup = 142 gms
anchovy	.14	—			
apples	.03	4	.3	7.5	2½″ dia = 150 gms
apple, dried	.135	—	3.	—	
apple juice	.03	—	.1	—	
apple sauce	.03	—	.2	—	1 cup = 239 gms
apricots	.07	—	.9	—	3 apricots = 114 gms
apricots, canned	.05	—	—	—	1 cup = 259 gms
apricots, dried	.25	—	5.0	—	
artichokes	.097	—	2.7	—	
asparagus	.16	38	2.3	4.2	1 cup = 11 spears = 175 gms
asparagus, canned	.06	—		—	
avocados	.42	19	2.2	22	½ avo. 4″ × 3″ = 123 gms
bacon, cured, raw	.125	141	9.1	.89	2 slices = 16 gms
banana, raw	.51	11	1.1	46	6″ × 1″ = 150 gms
barley, pearled	.26	114	11.4	2.3	1 cup = 203 gms
beans, kidney	.28	225	22	1.2	
beans, lima, raw	.17	134	8.4	1.3	1 cup = 160 gms
beans, lima, frozen	.15	—	—	—	
beans, lima, canned	.09	—			
beans, snap, raw	.08	28	1.9	2.9	1 cup = 125 gms
beans, snap, frozen	.07	—	—	—	
beans, snap, canned	.04	—	—	—	
beef, brain	.16	220	10.4	.73	3 oz = 85 gms
beef, heart	.29	403	16.8	.72	″ ″

—value not yet measured

Food	mg B₆ 100 gms	mg methionine / 100 gms	gm protein /100 gm	H-value ratio of B₆ to methionine x1000	standard portion
beef, kidneys	.39	307	15.4	1.3	" "
beef, liver	.70	463	19.7	1.5	" "
beef, round	.50	970	39	.52	" "
beef, tongue	.13	416	17.8	.31	" "
beer	.05	—	.5	—	1 cup = 240 gms
beets, peeled	.05	—	1.6	—	1 cup = 165 gms
beet greens	.10	37	2.2	2.7	
biscuits, baking powder	—	97	7.4	—	2½ " dia = 38 gms
brazil nuts	.17	941	14.3	.18	1 cup = 140 gms
bread, corn	—	27	3.4	—	
bread, French–Italian	.05	115	9.0	.43	1 slice = 23 gms
bread, protein	.17	196	10.8	.87	" "
bread, pumpernickel	.160	—	—	—	" "
bread, rye	.1	139	9.1	.72	1 slice = 23 gms
bread, white	.04	126	8.7	.32	" "
bread, whole wheat	.18	161	10.4	1.1	" "
brewers' yeast	4.0	2,500	46.5	1.6	1 tbs = 8 gms
broccoli, raw	.195	54	3.6	3.6	1 cup = 150 gms
broccoli, frozen	.150	—	—	—	
brussels sprouts, raw	.23	49	4.7	4.9	1 cup = 130 gms
brussels sprouts, frozen	.15	—	—	—	
buckwheat flour	.578	—	—	—	
bulgur, red	.225	268	11.1	.84	
butter	.003	21	.6	.14	1 pat = 7 gms; 1 cup = 227 gms
cabbage, red	.20	18	1.7	11	1 cup = 100 gms
cabbage, white	.16	12	1.3	13	1 cup = 100 gms
cake, angel	—	93	7.1	—	1/12 of 8" cake = 40 gms
cake, plain	.04	—	—	—	1/16 of 10" cake = 100 gms
calf, brain	.16	—	10.2	—	
calf, kidneys	.5	—	16.7	—	
calf, liver	1.2	447	19.2	2.7	
cantaloupes	.086	2	.7	43	½ melon 5" dia. = 385 gms
carrots	.15	10	1.2	15	1" × 5½" = 50 gms

Food	mg B₆ /100 gms	mg methionine/ 100 gms	gm protein /100 gm	H-value ratio of B₆ to methionine x1000	standard portion
carrots, canned	.03	—	—	—	
cashew nuts	—	330	17.2	—	1 cup = 135 gms
cauliflower	.21	54	2.7	3.9	1 cup = 120 gms
cauliflower, frozen	.19				
celery, raw	.06	16	1.1	3.7	1 stalk = 40 gms
cheese, American	.071	573	22.1	.12	
cheese, blue	.166	585	21.4	.28	
cheese, brie	.235	592	20.8	.40	
cheese, camembert	.227	565	19.8	.40	
cheese, cheddar	.07	653	25.0	.11	1″ cube = 17 gms
cheese, cottage, crmd.	.067	376	12.5	.18	1 cup = 235 gms; 1 tbs 15 gm
cheese, cottage, dry	.082	520	17.3	.16	1 cup = 235 gms 1 oz = 28 gms
cheese, cream	.047	181	7.5	.26	
cheese, parmesan	.091	958	35.7	.09	
cheese, Roquefort	.10	574	22.1	.17	
cheese, Swiss	.075	714	27.4	.11	
cherries, red, raw	.032	—	1.2	—	1 cup = 130 gms
chestnuts, fresh	.29	—	3.4	—	
chicken, flesh & skin	.5	537	20.6	.93	½ breast 76 gms drumstick 38 gms
chicken, liver	.8	520	21.0	1.5	
clams, raw	.08	—	10.5	—	3 oz = 85 gms
coconuts, fresh	.06	71	3.8	.85	1 cup = 97 gms
cod	.2	510	17.6	.39	
coffee	trace	—	—	—	
cola	—	—	—	—	
corn	.16	66	3.5	2.4	1 ear = 140 gms
corn, canned	.20	—	—	—	1 cup = 256 gms
cornflakes	.065	140	8.4	.46	1 cup = 28 gms
cornflour	.06	148	7.8	.41	
corn grits	.20	165	8.8	1.2	1 cup = 242 gms
corn meal, dry white	.35	153	7.8	2.3	1 cup = 145 gms
cornstarch	.005	—	.3	—	

Food	mg B$_6$ /100 gms	mg methionine / 100 gms	gm protein /100 gm	H-value ratio of B$_6$ to methionine x1000	standard portion
crab	.35	519	17.4	.67	
cranerries	.035	—	.4	—	
cream, heavy	.028	52	2.2	.54	1 tbs = 15 gms; 1 cup = 238 gms
cucumbers	.04	16	.9	2.5	7½″ × 2″ = 207 gms
currants, black, raw	.07	—	1.4	—	
dates	.15	26	2.2	5.8	1 cup = 178 gms
doughnut, plain	—	81	47	—	
duck	—	398	16.0	—	
eel, raw	.28	—	12.7	—	
eel, smoked	.15	—	—	—	
egg, chicken, white	.003	394	10.1	.008	1 white = 33 gms
egg, chicken, whole	.120	392	12.1	.31	1 egg = 50 gms
egg, chicken, yolk	.31	417	16.4	.74	1 yolk = 17 gms
egg, chicken, fried	.11	377	11.7	.28	
egg, hard-cooked	.11	392	12.1	.28	2 eggs = 100 gms
egg, chicken, powdered	.41	1481	45	.28	
egg, duck	.25	576	13.3	.43	
eggplant	—	6	1.2	—	
farina, flour	.067	148	11.4	.45	
fennel	.10	—	1.5	—	
figs, raw	.11	—	1.2	—	3, 1½″ = 114 gms
figs, dried	.18	—	4.3	—	1 fig 2″ × 1″ = 21 gms
flounder, raw	.17	434	15.8	.39	
frankfurter	.15	294	14	.51	1 frank = 51 gms
goose	.6	—	16.4	—	
goose liver	.9	—	17.0	—	
gooseberries	.012	—	.8	—	
grapefruit, raw	.034	—	.5	—	1 cup = 194 gms
grapefruit, canned	.02	—	—	—	
grapefruit juice, canned	.01	—	.4	—	1 cup = 246 grams
grapes, raw	.08	—	.6	—	1 cup = 160 grams
grape juice, fresh	.04	—	.2	—	1 cup = 254 gms

Food	mg B_6 / 100 gms	mg methionine / 100 gms	gm protein / 100 gm	H-value ratio of B_6 to methionine x1000	standard portion
grapenuts	—	140	10	—	
halibut, raw	.42	606	19.8	.69	
ham	.44	821	24.0	.54	3 oz = 85 gms
ham, cured	.27	—	—	—	1 2 oz slice = 57 gms
hazelnuts (filberts)	.54	120	11.7	4.5	
herring, raw	.37	502	17.3	.74	
herring, canned	.16	—	—	—	
herring, pickled	.12	—	—	—	
herring, smoked	.35	—	—	—	
honey	.01	—	.3	—	1 tbs = 21 gms
horseradish	.15	—	2.8	—	
ice cream, vanilla 16% fat	.036	70	2.79	.51	
ice cream, van. 10% fat	.046	91	3.61	.51	3½ oz = 62 gms
ice milk	.065	99	4.3	.66	1 cup = 187 gms
kale, raw	.30	38	4.2	7.9	1 cup = 110 gms
kale, frozen	.19	—	—	—	
kohlrabi, raw	.15	—	2.0	—	
lamb, raw	.275	538	18.5	.51	1 thick chop = 112 gms
lamb, braised	.181	—	—	—	
lamb, stewed	.231	—	—	—	
lamb, roasted	.201	—	—	—	
lemons, raw	.08	—	1.1	—	2½″ = 106 gms
lemon juice, fresh	.046	—	—	—	1 tbs = 15 gms; 1 cup = 246 gms
lentils, dried	.600	173	24.7	3.5	
lettue, head	.07	4	1.3	17.5	4″ dia Boston head = 220 gms
lime juice	.04	—	.3	—	1 cup = 246 gms
macaroni, dry	.064	370	12.5	.17	
mackeral, raw	.66	551	19.0	1.2	3 oz = 85 gms
mackeral, canned	.28	—	—	—	
mackeral, smoked	.41	—	—	—	

Food	mg B₆ /100 gms	mg methionine / 100 gms	gm protein /100 gm	H-value ratio of B₆ to methionine x1000	standard portion
masa harina	.51	—	9.4	—	—
masa trigo	.04	—	9.4	—	
milk, cow buttermilk	.034	123	3.3	.28	1 cup = 246 gms
milk, cow, evap. canned	.050	171	6.8	.29	1 cup = 252 gms
milk, cow, dry nonfat	.361	907	36.9	.40	
milk, cow, skimmed	.040	81	3.4	.49	
milk, cow, whole dry	.30	640	26.4	.47	
milk, cow, whole past.	.042	83	3.3	.51	1 cup = 244 gms
milk, goat, whole	.046	80	3.5	.58	
milk, human mature	.011	21	1.03	.52	
milk, mare	.03	—	2.1	—	
molasses	.20	—	—	—	
muffin, plain	—	143	7.7	—	
mushrooms, raw	.125	189	2.8	.66	
mushrooms, canned	.06	—	—	—	1 cup canned = 244 gms
noodles, egg dry	.088	216	12.8	.41	
noodles, egg cooked	—	70	4.1	—	1 cup = 160 gms
oat flakes	.75	—	13.8	—	
oatmeal, reg. dry	.21	—	16.2	—	
oatmeal, instnt, enriched	1.41	—	15.8	—	
okra, raw	.075	—	—	—	8 pods 3″ × ⅝″ = 85 gms
okra, frozen	.045	—	—	—	
oleomargarine	—	18	.71	—	1 cup = 227 gms; 1 pat = 7 gms
olives, green pckld	.02	—	1.4	—	4 med. = 16 gms
onions, raw	.13	—	1.5	—	2½″ dia = 110 gms
oranges, raw	.06	2.7	1.0	22	3″ dia = 210 gms
oranges, canned	.031	—	—	—	
orange juice, fresh	.040	—	—	—	1 cup = 248 gms
orange juice, canned	.035	—	—	—	
orange juice, frozen	.028	—	—	—	
oysters, raw	.05	—	9.0	—	
oysters, canned	.037	—	—	—	

Food	mg B₆ / 100 gms	mg methionine / 100 gms	gm protein /100 gm	H-value ratio of B₆ to methionine x1000	standard portion
pancake	—	146	7.1	—	1 cake = 27 gms
parsley	.16	18	3.6	8.9	1 tbs = 3.5 gms
parsnips	.1	—	1.7	—	
peaches, raw	.024	—	.4	—	1 peach = 114 gms
peaches, canned	.019	—	—	—	1 cup = 257 gms
peaches, frozen	.018	—	—	—	
peanuts, roasted	.3	265	26.2	1.1	1 cup = 140 gms
peanut butter	.33	265	27	1.2	1 tbs = 16 gms
pears, raw	.017	—	.5	—	3″ × 2½″ = 182 gms
pears, canned	.014	—	—	—	
peas, raw	.18	44	6.3	4.1	1 cup = 160 gms
peas, canned	.05	—	—	—	
peas, frozen	.13	—	—	—	
peas, split dried	.05	289	24.2	.17	
pecans	.19	150	9.2	1.3	1 cup = 108 gms; 1 tbs = 7.4 gms
peppers, green, raw	.26	16	1.2	16	1 pod = 62 gms
pineapples, raw	.09	—	.4	—	1 cup = 140 gms
pineapples, canned	.07	—	—	—	
pineapple juice, canned	.1	—	.4	—	1 cup = 249 gms
plantain	—	6	1.1	—	
plums, raw	.052	—	.7	—	2″ dia = 60 gms
plums, canned	.027	—	—	—	
pollen	.9	—	—	—	
popcorn, popped	.204	243	12.8	.84	1 cup = 14 gms
pork, cutlet or ribs	.48	220	12.0	2.2	2.3 oz = 66 gms
pork, heart	.43	421	16.9	1.0	
pork, kidneys	.55	334	16.3	1.6	
pork, liver	.85	463	20.1	1.8	
pork, tongue	.35	370	16.8	.95	
potatoes, raw	.25	25	2.1	10	1 potato = 99 gms
potatoes, canned	.10	—	—	—	
potato chips	.18	—	—	—	10 chips 2″ dia = 20 gms
pretzels	.019	—	—	—	
prunes, dried	.240	—	2.1	—	4 prunes = 32 gms
pumpkin, canned	.056	9	1.0	6.2	1 cup = 228 gms

Food	mg B$_6$ / 100 gms	mg methionine / 100 gms	gm protein /100 gm	H-value ratio of B$_6$ to methionine x1000	standard portion
rabbit, raw	.44	—	20.4	—	
radishes	.075	2	1.1	38	4 small, no tops = 40 gms
raisins, seedless	.24	—	2.5	—	1 cup = 160 gms
raspberries, raw	.06	—	1.2	—	1 cup = 123 gms
raspberries, frozen	.038	—	—	—	
rhubarb, raw	.03	—	.5	—	1 cup = 272 gms
rice, brown, raw	.55	136	7.5	4.0	
rice, white dry polished	.15	—	—	—	
rice, white precooked	.034	—	—	—	
rice, puffed cereal	.075	—	—	—	1 cup = 14 gms
rolls, hard white	.035	127	8.3	.28	1 roll = 38 gms
royal jelly	1.0	—	—	—	
rutabaga	.10	—	—	—	
rye flour, light	.09	149	9.7	.60	
rye flour, whole	.30	182	11.4	1.65	
salmon, raw	.70	655	25.2	1.1	
salmon, canned	.30	—	—	—	3 oz = 85 gms
salmon, salted, smoked	.70	—	—	—	
sardines, canned	.18	597	20.6	.30	
sauerkraut, canned	.18	—	—	—	1 cup = 235
sausage, salami	.123	—	—	—	8 .1" slices = 227 gms
shrimp, raw	.10	545	18.7	.18	
shrimp, canned	.06	—	—	—	
soybeans, dried raw	.81	512	34.1	1.6	
soy flour, high-fat	.635	620	41	1.0	
spaghetti, dry	.064	190	12.6	.34	
spinach, raw	.28	54	3.2	5.2	1 cup = 180 gms
spinach, frozen	.19	—	—	—	
squash, raw summer	.082	—	—	—	1 cup = 210 gms
squash, raw winter	.154	—	—	—	1 cup = 205 gms
strawberries, raw	.055	—	.7	—	1 cup = 149 gms
strawberries, frozen	.043	—	—	—	
sugar, white	0	—	—	—	
sunflower seed kernel	1.250	—	—	—	
sweet potato, raw	.218	31	1.7	7.0	5" × 2" = 110 gms
sweet potato, canned	.066	—	—	—	

Food	mg B₆ 100 gms	mg methionine / 100 gms	gm protein /100 gm	H-value ratio of B₆ to methionine x1000	standard portion
tangerines	.07	—	.8	—	2½″ dia = 114 gms
tomatoes, raw	.1	8	1.1	12.5	2″ × 2½″ = 150 gms
tomatoes, canned	.09	—	—	—	
tomato juice, canned	.19	—	.9	—	1 cup = 246 gms
tomato puree	.18	12	2.0	15	
tortilla, yellow corn	.073	93	5	.79	
tuna, raw	.90	—	—	—	
tuna, canned	.425	1062	24.0	.40	3 oz = 85 gms
turkey	—	558	20.1		
turnips, raw	.09	11	1.0	8.2	1 cup = 155 gms
turnip greens	.26	54	3.0	4.8	1 cup = 145 gms
veal, rib, raw	.43	631	23.5	.68	3 oz = 85 gms
veal, braised	.35	—	—	—	
veal, roasted	.28	—	—	—	
veal, stewed	.35	—	—	—	
vegetable fat	0	—	0	—	
vinegar	.001	—	—	—	
walnuts	.73	306	14.9	2.4	1 cup = 100 gms; 1 tbs = 8 gms
watermelon	.068	—	.5	—	1 ″ wedge 4″ × 8″ = 925 gms
wheat flakes	.292	144	12.2	2.0	1 oz = 28 gms
wheat flour, white	.06	136	10.5	.44	1 cup = 110 gms
wheat flour, whole wheat	.34	200	13.3	1.7	1 cup = 120 gms
wheat germ	1.15	430	26.6	2.7	1 cup = 68 gms
wheat, shredded	.244	137	10	1.8	
whey, fluid	.042	14	.76	3.0	
wine	.09	—	.7	—	
yeast, bakers' dry active	2.00	—	—	—	
yoghurt, plain	.032	102	3.47	.31	1 cup = 246 gms.

Table 2

AMOUNT OF VITAMIN B₆ LOST

	Frozen	Canned	Final Cooking
Fish and Seafood	17%	49%	46%
Meats and Poultry	—	43%	46%
Dairy Products	—	16%	—
Root Vegetables	—	63%	—
Legume Vegetables	56%	77%	25%
Green Vegetables	37%	57%	25%
Fruit and Fruit Juice	16%	38%	—
Pasta Products	—	—	50%

Table 2 shows the average loss of vitamin B_6 in preparing foods. For a particular food, for example a seafood, if it is frozen and then cooked, the amount of vitamin B_6 in the product as eaten, will be reduced, first, 17% by the freezing process and then, the remaining amount will be reduced an additional 46% in the final cooking. For items with dashes, the loss of vitamin B_6 has not yet been determined (from Lushbough et al. 1959; Schroeder 1971; CRC 1972).

COMPARISON OF DIETS: H-VALUE

With the tables at hand, we can compute the daily intake of vitamin B_6 and methionine for a variety of diets. For any particular food we find its content of vitamin B_6 and methionine contents in Table 1: If that food has been canned, commercially frozen and/or cooked, we then reduce the vitamin B_6 content by the percentages shown in Table 2.

From the homocysteine theory, we know that it isn't merely the amount of vitamin B_6 that is critical, but the amount of vitamin B_6 compared to the amount of methionine. A good rule of thumb for deciding if a diet is adequate is to determine the ratio of vitamin B_6 to methionine and then multiply it by 1000. If the ensuing number, which we call the "H-value," is less than 1, the diet is deficient. If it is greater than 1, it is generally adequate. All the known human populations (from Bedouins to

Eskimos) whose members have low levels of arteriosclerosis have diets with H-value greater than 1. In Table 1 we have computed the H-value of each food. It is quite clear that most animal products, especially after cooking, have H-values less than 1. Vegetable products tend to have H-values greater than 1.

Let us examine and compare three different diets: (1) an ordinary American diet; (2) a low cholesterol/high protein diet (along lines suggested by the Scarsdale Medical Diet); (3) a diet designed to increase vitamin B$_6$ intake relative to methionine intake.

Ordinary American Diet

	amount (grams)	vitamin B$_6$ (mg) raw	as eaten	methionine (mg)
Breakfast				
orange	210	.13	.13	6
2 eggs, fried	100	.12	.11	377
3 strips bacon	24	.03	.02	34
coffee	220	0	0	0
sugar	8	0	0	0
Lunch				
⅓ lb. hamburger	113	.56	.26	1090
white roll	38	0	.01	48
french fries	100	.25	.20	25
cola	248	0	0	0
apple	150	.05	.05	0
Dinner				
6 oz. beefsteak	170	.85	.46	1650
green peas, cooked frozen	80	.10	.08	35
hash brown potatoes	100	.25	.20	25
cottage cheese	60	.04	.04	226
lettuce salad	55	.04	.04	3
ice cream	62	.03	.03	56
Totals			1.63	3,575

We see that this day's meals contain 1.63 mg of vitamin B_6, less even than the RDA of 2 mg. That is of some concern, but since the homocysteine theory is concerned with the ratio of vitamin B_6 intake to methionine intake, let us compute the overall H-value for the day:

$$\text{H-value for day's meals} = (B_6 \div \text{methionine}) \times 1000 = \frac{1.63}{3575} \times 1000 = .46$$

We can see that the H-value is significantly less than 1. Unfortunately, this is typical of most American diets.

Let us now examine a popular diet that is low in cholesterol and high in protein:

Low Cholesterol/High Protein Diet—from Scarsdale Medical Diet (Tarnower and Baker 1980)

	amount (grams)	vitamin B_6 (mg) raw	as eaten	methionine (mg)	protein (grams)
Breakfast					
½ grapefruit	130	.04	.04	4	1
protein bread (slice)	23	—	.04	45	2.5
coffee/tea	—	—	—	—	—
Lunch					
cold cuts:					
chicken	50	.25	.14	270	10
beef (lean)	50	.25	.14	485	20
broiled tomato	150	.15	.13	12	1.5
coffee/diet soda	—	—	—	—	—
Dinner					
broiled halibut, 8 oz.	225	.95	.51	1370	45
cooked zucchini	105	.08	.06	4	0.5
lettuce head	220	.15	.15	9	3
protein bread (slice)	23	—	.04	45	2.5
½ grapefruit	130	.04	.04	4	1
Totals			1.29	2248	87.0

As in diet 1, the vitamin B_6 intake is less than 2 mg for the day. The H-value is:

$$\text{H-value for day} = (B_6 \div \text{methionine}) \times 1000 = \frac{1.29}{2248} = .57$$

Again, the H-value is significantly lower than 1. So we see that a diet designed to be low in cholesterol is not necessarily adequate from the perspective of the homocysteine theory. Let us now examine a diet in which we select foods with the goal of significantly increasing the overall H-value for the day's meals:

High H-Value Diet

	amount (grams)	vitamin B_6 (mg) raw	as eaten	methionine (mg)	protein (grams)
Breakfast					
orange juice, 1 cup	248	.10	.10	6	2.5
cornflakes 1 oz.	28	.50	.50	140	2.3
banana	150	.75	.75	16	1.6
milk (1 cup)	244	.10	.10	200	8.0
Lunch					
raw carrot	50	.08	.08	5	0.6
peanut butter	48	.17	.17	135	13.0
whole wheat bread (2 slices)	46	.08	.08	70	4.8
apple	150	.04	.04	6	0.5
Dinner					
guacamole (½ avocado)	108	.50	.50	24	2.7
chicken, 3 oz.	85	.42	.22	460	18.5
potato, baked	99	.25	.20	25	2.1
broccoli, cooked	150	.30	.23	80	5.4
angel cake	—	—	—	40	2.8
coffee	—	—	—	—	—
	—	—	—	—	—
Totals			2.97	1207	64.8

In this diet we have attained both higher intake of vitamin B_6 and lower intake of methionine. It has a moderate amount of protein and there is no necessity for restriction of the types of food eaten. The only limitations we imposed are concerned with quantity of foods high in methionine.

$$\text{H-value} = (B_6 \div \text{methionine}) \times 1000 = \frac{2.97}{1207} \times 1000 = 2.46$$

The H-value is more than four times that of the high protein/low cholesterol diet.

AMERICAN DIETS

In the above example we have devised a day's meals which are reasonably low in methionine and exceeds the RDA of 2 to 2.2 mg per day of vitamin B_6 for non-pregnant adults and 2.6 mg per day of vitamin B_6 for pregnant women, but it is difficult to devise a nutritionally adequate diet that consistently contains such amounts. A most graphic example of this comes from the work done by Aurora Mangay Chung and her colleagues at Vanderbilt and Tulane universities, who designed a set of well-balanced meals in which cost was no object. These meals were relentlessly diverse and planned along guidelines found in such books as the *Betty Crocker Picture Cookbook* and the *Good Housekeeping Cookbook*. Any energetic newlywed with time, love, and money to spare, access to an American supermarket, and no taste for the exotic, could produce these three-a-day feasts. We have reproduced on pp. 148–149 the menu for one week's meals.

What is surprising is that even with these wonderful meals, the average daily vitamin B_6 intake would be merely 2 mg (and the H-value estimated for the whole week's diet a mere 0.43). And who eats this way? Very few contemporary Americans. Professor Judy Driskell's study showed that in the actual diets of young adults, 64 percent of the males and 92 percent of the females took in less than 2 mg per day of vitamin B_6. In addition, 17 percent of the males and 35 percent of the females had less than 1 mg per day of vitamin B_6. In Cleary's study of pregnant women eating normally, "Only one of 26 subjects consumed the [then] RDA of 2.5 mg pyridoxine daily. Eighteen subjects ingested 1.9 mg or less." In a survey of American school lunches it was found that more than half did not meet even the modest government recommendations for vitamin B_6.

If the recommended daily allowance for vitamin B_6 were doubled or tripled, as several nutritionists have proposed, one would be hard pressed to find anyone in the United States (other than queen bees; see Table 1 for royal jelly) that would have an adequate dietary intake of vitamin B_6 without supplement.

One Week's Menu of High Cost Diets

				Day			
	1	2	3	4	5	6	7
				Breakfast			
	Grapefruit with cherry Scrambled eggs Bacon Muffins Jelly Butter Milk Coffee	Tangerine juice Fried egg Country sliced ham Biscuits Preserves Butter Milk Coffee	Orange juice Pancakes with syrup Canadian bacon Coffee Milk	Grapefruit juice Cornflakes with milk Scrambled eggs Sausage Jelly Muffins Butter Coffee	Grapefruit with cherry Maltomeal with milk Poached egg Toast Butter Jelly Coffee	Orange juice Waffles with syrup Link sausage Coffee Milk	Tangerine juice French toast with syrup Canadian bacon Coffee Milk
				Lunch			
	Cream of asparagus soup with crackers Tuna salad sandwich with relishes Potato chips Lemon meringue pie	Pizza pie (pepperoni) Italian salad (lettuce, cucumber, egg, tomatoes, green pepper, spinach)	Mixed grill (lamb chop, bacon, sweetbread, tomatoes, pineapple, banana) Biscuits Butter Tapioca pudding	Shrimp salad bowl (eggs, shrimps, celery, pickles) Potato chips Cherry pie a la mode Milk	Oyster stew Toasted cheese and bacon sandwich Relishes White cake with raisin and almond garnish	Chef's salad dinner plate (cheese, bacon, egg, celery, green pepper, carrots, and lettuce) Ritz® crackers Orange	Turkey pot pie Tomatoes and cucumber salad Apple pie with cheese Milk Coffee

		Milk		Dinner	monds Milk	shortcake Milk	cracker crust Coffee
Carrot and celery curls	Chilled fruit cocktail		Potato snap-pies	V-8 juice cocktail	Cocktail anchovies with Ritz crackers	Stuffed celery	Shrimp hors d'oeuvres
Fried chicken	Seafood platter (shrimps, scallops, oysters)		Liver and onions	Baked ham with fruit sauce	Fresh pork tenderloin	Roast fillet of beef	Broiled T-bone steak
Mashed potatoes	French fries		Paprika potatoes	Mashed potatoes	Mashed sweet potatoes with marshmallow	Mashed potatoes	French fries
Buttered broccoli*	Carrots*		Asparagus*	Green peas*	Broccoli*	Buttered green beans	Buttered green peas* with mushrooms
Apple, grape, and celery salad	Head lettuce salad		Rolls	Pineapple, cabbage, and marshmallow salad	Pear and cheese salad	Fresh fruit salad	Tossed salad
Hot rolls	Hot rolls		Butter	Rolls	Orange sherbet with chocolate chip cookies	Angel food cake with fudge sauce	Hot rolls
Butter	Butter		Cole slaw	Butter	Coffee	Coffee	Butter
pumpkin pie with whipped cream	Strawberry sundae		Vanilla macaroon cupcake	Pecan fudge devil's food cake			Cherry vanilla ice cream
Coffee	Coffee		Coffee	Coffee			Coffee

*Frozen A week's menus that are designed to be nutritionally adequate overall and provide 2 mg per day of vitamin B_6. Very few people regularly eat this way and it is achieved by eating foods containing large amounts of methionine (hence the H-value is quite low) (from Chung et al. 1961).

149

CHAPTER 8
Dietary Implications of the Theory

ACCORDING TO THE HOMOCYSTEINE THEORY, our diets should contain moderate levels of methionine (which means moderate protein intake), coupled with sufficient vitamin B$_6$. Vitamin B$_6$ intake should satisfy the NAS–NRC criterion (although not the NAS–NRC chosen RDA) to "afford a margin sufficiently above average physiological requirements to cover variations among practically all individuals in the general population."

Taking into consideration the material in Chapters 6 and 7, we propose that protein intake for relatively sedentary adults should be 50 grams daily (just under two ounces) for a 150-pound person. People of different weight should consume proportionally greater or lesser amounts of protein. We obviously require protein in our diet but the homocysteine theory shows that excessive protein is not healthy since it will lead to excessive methionine intake.

A reasonable vitamin B$_6$ intake should be 10 to 25 mg per day depending on individual conditions (people who are old, pregnant, lactating, using oral contraceptives, consuming large amounts of protein, or having vascular problems should take amounts at the higher end of the range). Megadoses do not seem useful, since there is a plateau above which the body does not seem to utilize the vitamin and rapidly excretes the excess.

Protein intake of 50 grams per day is not meager. The current RDA for men is 70 grams and for women, 50 grams. Those who now eat large amounts of protein can make commonsense reductions, such as eating one hamburger instead of two and drinking smaller glasses of milk. A small hamburger contains about 20 grams of protein; a large egg contains six grams of protein; an eight ounce glass of whole milk contains approximately seven grams of protein.

One problem that arises from our suggestions is that it is quite difficult to select foods that simultaneously yield a daily intake of vitamin B_6, on the order of 10 mg, while avoiding large quantities of protein. One solution is to take vitamin B_6 supplements. We are reluctant to suggest supplements, since they would seem to add to the predilection to overmedicate that afflicts our society. There is something unattractive about the proposition—take a potion and be cured. Our distaste is perhaps a residue of our Puritan ethic: To be really cured, one must work hard.

However, logically, we see vitamin B_6 supplementation as a straightforward and reasonable approach. Vitamin B_6 is not a foreign substance, like most medications, since it is already in our food. It also is quite safe.

SAFETY OF PYRIDOXINE

The safety of vitamin B_6 should not be claimed offhand. Any advice to change one's dietary regimen should meet the Hippocratic dictum—"Do no harm." We have to be *sure* that vitamin B_6 is a safe compound in the quantities that we suggest.

In fact, wide investigation by many laboratories supports the claim. There is almost universal agreement that vitamin B_6 has no toxic effect unless extremely large doses are ingested. In the latest edition of Goodman and Gilman's *The Pharmacological Basis of Therapeutics,* a virtual bible of medical practice, Dr. Paul Greengard of the Department of Pharmacology of Yale University writes: "Pyridoxine elicits no outstanding pharmacodynamic actions after either oral or intravenous administration. Large doses in the range of 3 to 4 gms/kg [grams per kilogram] produce convulsions and death in animals, but lower doses can be given daily without any obvious effects."

An adult weighing 150 pounds (approximately 68 kg) would have to eat about a half pound (about 200 gms) to reach the dose level associated with serious toxic effects. Even ingestion of a half pound of table salt would be toxic. For a 150 pound person, a dose of 10 mg is 20,000 times smaller than the "large dose." We are indeed discussing the use of very small quantities of vitamin B_6.

OVERDOSE OF VITAMIN B_6?

Warnings still circulate that intake of 50 mg of pyridoxine daily (a dose about four thousand times less than Greengard's "large dose") of vitamin B_6 taken by pregnant women can be detrimental to their offspring. The warnings are without merit and originated in the 1950s as a consequence of the S-M-A liquid milk concentrate emergency discussed in the previous chapter. We described how convulsions in infants were traced to a milk concentrate that contained too low a vitamin B_6 concentration. The discovery that vitamin B_6 deficiency could lead to such a serious consequence made pediatricians keen to ensure that pregnant women and infants took adequate amounts of the vitamin. This, in turn, led to an unexpected development. Dr. Andrew Hunt and his colleagues at the Children's Hospital in Philadelphia presented a case in 1954 that purported to show that because a pregnant woman took large doses of pyridoxine, her infant daughter had become addicted to pyridoxine and had developed a pyridoxine dependency (equivalent to a narcotic dependency).

During her first pregnancy, the woman took no pyridoxine supplement and delivered a normal infant. During her second pregnancy, she received pyridoxine supplements; the infant suffered convulsions, then died. Again, during her third pregnancy, the woman received pyridoxine supplements; this infant also suffered convulsions, but survived. The infant, who became retarded, could be kept convulsion-free, it was found, with large daily doses of vitamin B_6. Dr. Hunt and his colleagues concluded that the infant had become dependent on pyridoxine in the same way that infants of alcoholic mothers become alcohol-dependent.

This single case was extensively quoted. It seemed to contain a simple lesson: Too much vitamin B_6 can be dangerous. But, although the argument was logically consistent, later experimental tests eventually showed it was wrong. Three years later, Dr. Hunt himself experimentally followed up his earlier work. He knew that when nursing rats are given a pyridoxine-deficient diet, their offspring, like human infants, develop serious symptoms of vitamin B_6 deficiency. Also, like human infants, they lose weight and frequently convulse, starting at about three weeks of age. With this as background, Hunt took pregnant rats and divided them into two groups. During the first half of pregnancy he gave one group massive doses of pyridoxine mixed in their daily ration; the other group received the usual diet. After delivery, the nursing mothers in both groups received diets devoid of vitamin B_6. Hunt's hypothesis predicted that there should be a higher incidence of convulsions in the litters of mothers given massive vitamin B_6 doses during pregnancy since these rats would be the ones to develop the pyridoxine dependency. "No such correlation, however, was observed in any of the trials," wrote Hunt. "Indeed, if there were any positive results they were in the opposite direction, with the offspring of the experimental group having a slightly better weight gain than those in the control group. Experimental evidence in support of the hypothesis that abnormal need for vitamin B_6 could be related to overdose of this substance during pregnancy is therefore lacking."

So Hunt's hypothesis of what happened to the patient at Children's Hospital and her daughter was not validated experimentally. Further work has revealed that some individuals suffer congenital abnormalities of vitamin B_6 metabolism. Dr. Hunt and his colleagues apparently came upon such a situation with the woman's second and third offspring by coincidence. In 1966 the American Academy of Pediatrics Committee on Nutrition issued a report entitled "Vitamin B_6 Requirements in Man" (Lowe et al. 1966). They reviewed the literature and concluded that vitamin B_6 dependency "is probably inherited as a recessive condition." They knew of Hunt's original work and his follow-up experiments and observed that "to date, there has been no report of deleterious effects associated with daily oral ingestion of large doses of vitamin B_6 (.2 to 1 gm per day [2 gm = 200 mg]."

Despite both Hunt's retraction and the AAP study, Hunt's first paper is still cited as a caveat against high doses of pyridoxine. In 1976 Drs. J.Y. Levy and P. Bach y Rita wrote a book, *Vitamins—Their Use and Abuse,* in response to the recent spate of claims for various vitamin therapies. The authors, in an effort to act responsibly, introduced some elements of caution. One of the topics discussed was vitamin B_6 supplements for pregnant women. They wrote, "Babies born of mothers on high doses of vitamin B_6 may have excessively high B_6 requirements, and if these are not met, serious problems could develop in the infant." For verification of this claim they referred to a secondary reference which cited Hunt's original paper. Levy and Bach y Rita obviously did not know of Hunt's later retraction (19 years prior to the publication of their book) or of the report of the American Academy of Pediatrics (ten years prior to the publication of their book). The net effect of this was that while ostensibly taking the responsible position, they had not done their homework and were in fact perpetuating an incorrect myth. As far as is known, 10 to 25 mg of vitamin B_6 daily is safe.

DANGERS OF VITAMIN B_6 IN NURSING MOTHERS?

Dr. Leonard B. Greentree (1979) suggested in a letter to the *New England Journal of Medicine* that even small doses of vitamin B_6 could inhibit lactation by inhibiting the milk-producing hormone prolactin. However, Drs. E. del Pozo and R. Brun del Re (1979) of Universitäts—Frauenklinik in Basel, Switzerland, subsequently wrote that they found that even administration of 600 mg daily to 11 postpartum women failed to suppress either prolactin or lactation.

COMPETITIVE EFFECTS?

Several popular texts also warn against vitamin B$_6$ supplements on the basis of so-called competitive effects. The claim is that if only vitamin B$_6$ is increased, without equivalent increases in other B vitamins, this could lead to deficiencies in the other B vitamins. In *Let's Eat Right to Keep Fit*, Adele Davis writes, "It appears that all B vitamins work together; this cooperation is called the synergistic action of the B vitamins. The taking of one or more B vitamins increases the need for the others not supplied, probably because any one B vitamin alone can increase the activity of each body cell." In *Nutrition Almanac*, J.D. Kirschmann writes that the B vitamins "are so interrelated in function that large doses of any one of them may be therapeutically valueless or cause a deficiency of others. For example, if extra B$_6$ is taken in 50 mg potencies, it is important that a complete B complex accompany it."

Neither book cites primary scientific sources, and as far as we know there is no support for the claim that vitamin B$_6$ in large amounts antagonizes intake of other B vitamins. Indeed, the available evidence is in the other direction. For instance, Drs. A.R. Morrison and Herbett P. Sarett of the Department of Nutritional and Biochemical Research, Mead Johnson and Company, performed tests (on growing rats) to determine the interrelationship of various B vitamins, including vitamin B$_6$. To see if excess levels of one B vitamin would worsen the effects of deficiency in the other three, they administered excess levels of only one of four B vitamins while keeping the animals deficient in the other three. Their conclusion: "No adverse effects of high levels of . . . pyridoxine or [two other B vitamins] were observed."

ABNORMAL ELECTROENCEPHALOGRAMS?

We have found a single citation claiming an abnormal electroencephalographic (EEG) effect as a consequence of large but not huge vitamin B$_6$ supplements. It is an abstract of only a few lines and of dubious merit, but since we propose supplementing diets with 10 to 25 mg of pyridoxine, it is important to present any potential deleterious effects. Dr. J.E. Canham and his colleagues reported that eight normal adult males (27–43 years of age) with normal electroencephalograms were given normal diets supplemented with 200 mg per day of pyridoxine for 33 days. Eight days after cessation of the supplementation, three of the eight subjects had abnormal EEGs manifested by "low voltage with slowing of the frequency." Clinical electroencephalographers generally do not use low voltage and slowing of frequency as signs of significant brain disorders. Low voltage is often associated with technical problems in making contact between electrodes and the skull. Slowing of EEG frequency is generally related to the "mood" of the subject and occurs frequently in normal people. Thus, the claim is difficult to assess without a rather complete idea of the extent of slowing and diminution of the amplitude. The possibility of an effect of vitamin B_6 on the brain remains open (the study does not rule it out), but the abstract does not prove that such an effect exists and the authors never followed up their brief comments with a complete paper.

CONTRAINDICATION—LEVODOPA

There is one condition where supplements of pyridoxine are unwise and should be proscribed: patients with Parkinson's disease who are being treated with the drug levodopa. The characteristic shaking symptoms of Parkinson's disease are associated with degeneration of certain nerve fibers in the brain, which normally release the substance dopamine. The therapeutic approach to the disease is to increase the amount of dopamine in the brain (Franz 1975). A patient with Parkinson's disease cannot simply eat foods rich in dopamine since there is a barrier preventing the passage of dopamine from blood to brain. To get around this, the patient eats another substance, levodopa (or L-dopa), which can pass from blood to brain, and gives rise to dopamine (Leon et al. 1971). Once in the brain, levodopa is converted to dopamine by an enzyme and there is rapid remission of the Parkinson's symptoms. This enzyme, which exists in both the blood and the brain, needs vitamin B_6 as a coenzyme to work. If extra pyridoxine is available in the blood, levodopa will be converted more efficiently to dopamine in the bloodstream and little levodopa will be left over to go from blood to brain.

MEGADOSES OF VITAMIN B_6

Although we see no need for large intakes of vitamin B_6, it is worthwhile knowing the effects of such a regimen. A 1973 study dealing with this subject had the intriguing title "High Pyridoxine Diet in the Rat: Possible Implications for Megavitamin Therapy." Large doses of pyridoxine were given to rats to determine the vitamin's effect on metabolism and to test for toxicity. Phyllis Cohen and colleagues at the N.Y. Institute for Basic Research in Mental Retardation and Mount Sinai Hospital in New York found that rats on higher pyridoxine diets consumed the same amount of food as controls but had 20 percent greater body weight and 40 percent greater liver weight. The researchers presumed there was "an increase in food-utilization efficiency in rats fed the high pyridoxine diet." They said that the amount of pyridoxine ingested by the experimental group would be equivalent to a daily dose of 1.5 to 2.0 grams for a 70 kg man. This is indeed a large intake, about 150 times the suggested 10 mg a day. Biochemically, the group found "no significant differences in the concentrations of any of the amino acids measured in any of the tissues studied."

The experimenters seemed displeased by the lack of toxic effects from so large a pyridoxine intake, for they ended on a note of pique: "Little comfort can be taken in the fact that the rats on the high pyridoxine diet grew larger than the pair-fed controls, since it is well known that overnutrition is associated with decreased longevity." For this assertion, they cited an earlier work by R.A. McCance who wrote in 1962: "However beneficial a high plane of nutrition may be during growth, if it leads to obesity in an adult man it shortens the length of time he is likely to live to enjoy it." It is not clear that high pyridoxine levels in humans lead to obesity. So it is misleading to claim that "overnutrition" *per se* will decrease longevity. We *do* take comfort from the fact that Dr. Cohen and her colleagues obtained such normal results in rats on large doses of pyridoxine, levels as we say, the equivalent to 150 times greater than the 10 mg a day we have suggested.

AVAILABILITY OF SUPPLEMENTS

Given the safety of vitamin B_6, it seems reasonable to explore ways in which to assure adequate intake. In 1964 Dr. Henry Borsook of the California Institute of Technology suggested that "there is a strong case for increasing the B_6 in the food supply. . . . the only feasible method of augmenting the B_6 in the United States diet is by adding to the enrichment formula of flour and bread. . . . In general, there is less B_6 (on a milligram basis) than riboflavin [vitamin B_2]. Riboflavin is a mandatory component of the flour and bread enrichment formula because riboflavin in the American diet is, otherwise, too low. The B_6 requirement is, if anything, higher than the riboflavin requirement. If enrichment with riboflavin is called for, then the call is even stronger for enrichment with B_6."

Since pyridoxine is heat-stable, baking flour enriched with pyridoxine will not adversely affect its vitamin B_6 content. It is important to remember that flour is currently enriched with three B vitamins, niacin, thiamin, and riboflavin. Thus, it is not a radical step to add vitamin B_6 to the flour. (In fact, Canada already requires enriched bread to contain .28 mg of vitamin B_6 per 100 grams.) Such common products as white bread, hamburger rolls, and tacos could thereby supply significant quantities of vitamin B_6. In the latest available report, listed in the Encyclopedia of Chemical Technology, the price of pyridoxine hydrochloride was $30 per kg (Harris et al. 1968). This means that if every person in the United States were supplemented with 10 mg of vitamin B_6 each day, the yearly bill for pyridoxine for the entire U.S. population would come to approximately $22 million, about 10 cents per person per year!

A mandated supplementation of pyridoxine in flour products could lead to a civil liberties question, as well as a nutritional issue. It is an extension of the general debate whether it is right to supplement foods at all. We take a bit of a waffling position on the matter: Enrichment of foods has been permitted and it seems reasonable that if supplementation is allowed, it should be made as effective as possible.

People within the National Research Council-National Academy of Sciences, the group that establishes the RDA, are becoming concerned about deficits of vitamin B_6 (and other components) in American diets. In 1974, ten years after Borsook's suggestion, the panel of the Committee on Food Standards and Fortification Policy of the Food and Nutrition Board NAS–NRC proposed (Bauernfeind and Miller 1978) that "(1) since cereal grain products constitute 26 percent of the daily caloric intake, (2) since they are suitable carriers for the addition of nutrients to the diet because of their broad usage by almost everyone in the United States, and (3) since there is evidence of potential risk of deficiency of vitamin A, thiamin, riboflavin, niacin, vitamin B_6, folacin, iron, calcium, magnesium, and zinc among significant segments of the population, cereal grain products be nutrified with these nutrients."

It is interesting that the panel acknowledged the "potential risk of deficiency" of vitamin B_6 and other compounds, although they do not spell out the risk. They suggested fortifying cereal grain products to a pyridoxine level of 2 mg per lb. This is a quite small supplement and is not mandatory. Enrichment with pyridoxine has nevertheless been carried out since 1976 by some of the major producers of dry breakfast cereals such as Kellogg's and General Mills. They have added 0.5 mg pyridoxine per one-ounce serving of their standard products such as Rice Krispies and Wheaties (four times the NAS–NRC panel's recommended supplement). Such an industry decision is a step in the right direction. Pyridoxine is still not added to "natural cereals," nor to most enriched bread (such as Wonder Bread) made from "enriched flour" which *is* fortified with iron and three B vitamins.

Until the day when food is sufficiently enriched (or we start eating like Eskimos or Bedouins), individuals can supplement their diet simply by taking vitamin B_6 in the form of pyridoxine hydrochloride tablets. These are available over-the-counter in most pharmacies in concentrations ranging from 10 mg to 100 mg per tablet. The larger dose tablets can be broken up into smaller pieces and still supply adequate vitamin B_6.

As we mentioned earlier, our suggested RDA for vitamin B_6 of between 10 and 25 mg a day raises the requirement beyond what can be practically obtained in typical American diets. There is a precedent for such a course of action. In the 1974 edition of the Recommended Daily Dietary Allowance of the Food and Nutrition Board, NAS–NRC, the RDA for iron for pregnant women had been set so high that "the use of supplemental iron is recommended." At this date, supplements of vitamin B_6 would seem in order.

So, we suggest that vitamin B_6 is very safe and the RDA should be raised to between 10 and 25 mg, depending on individual conditions. At the present time the simplest way to obtain sufficient vitamin B_6 is through vitamin supplements. People should also adjust their intake of protein to the order of 50 grams per day for a 150-pound adult.

And we suggest strongly that anyone contemplating any changes in diet should first consult with a physician.

CHAPTER 9

The Homocysteine Theory, Medicine, and Society

SEVERAL YEARS AGO an epidemiologist came to the Arteriosclerosis Center at our university to give a seminar on the topic "Arteriosclerosis in Israel." As we pointed out in Chapter 1, Israel has been an important center of epidemiological studies because of the diversity of the population and major differences in incidence of coronary disease. The epidemiologist had reams of data summarized on about 40 slides. He showed the relative importance of many different risk factors. The usual dietary possibilities were mentioned: cholesterol, fatty acids, total fat, protein, carbohydrates, and sugar, among others. Nondietary factors were also investigated: psychological profiles, including marital status, supportiveness of mate, and general stress. Even exercise was discussed. Our heads were saturated with numbers and tables.

Through the mass of data several points could be distilled. Individually, each of the dietary factors had little impact on coronary risk and only one of the nondietary factors substantially influenced risk—exercise. Most important, one area stood out by its absence. Despite the massive array of risk factors studied and blood components measured, the investigators did not look at dietary intake of methionine or vitamin B_6, nor did they measure serum homocysteine or serum pyridoxal phospate.

During the discussion period that followed, we asked: What about homocysteine? The epidemiologist had little to say since his group hadn't been concerned with the topic. But one of the clinicians in the audience who worked at the Arteriosclerosis

Center did respond. Yes, he knew of the work of "Killy" McCully (they had been classmates in medical school and McCully worked across the river and had given talks at the center). He didn't see how homocysteine could be important in development of arteriosclerosis since homocystinurics have a considerably higher incidence of thromboses than other people with severe arteriosclerosis, so a different process must be at work.

We didn't argue the point then. Now we would respond by suggesting that while high concentrations of homocysteine might lead to a proportionally higher amount of thromboses, this in no way eliminates the possibility that homocysteine could also be the critical factor in arteriosclerosis. Certainly, the pathology that develops in the arterial wall after homocysteine exposure matches the pathology of arteriosclerosis. In addition, a relatively low level of serum homocysteine could cause arteriosclerosis over the long run, yet not be expected to cause a particularly high incidence of thromboses, whereas a high level of serum homocysteine could cause both a high incidence of thromboses and arteriosclerosis. Different effects do not necessarily scale up evenly.

In any case, it was instructive to see that the theory was not taken seriously. The clinician's answer was glib. Even a physician interested in risk factors should at least be curious to see what is the risk of coronary disease associated with homocystinemia. If a risk could be demonstrated, then most clinicians would agree the relationship between dietary components and serum homocysteine should be explored.

We have come to believe that homocysteine is not currently being studied because the prevailing ideas about risk factors and the importance of cholesterol—whether right or wrong—nonetheless serve the important purpose of tying together the enormous amount of information that has been compiled over the years. It has already become a gigantic task to sift research material on the currently accepted factors. People in the field have followed their instincts and discarded some data and not bothered to pursue what seem like obscure paths in a search for tiny clues. We saw earlier in our hypothetical model for trying to establish a recommended dietary allowance for vitamin B$_6$ that we could choose an unlimited number of variables to correlate with vitamin B$_6$-dependent compounds. But there was no pressing need.

And many clinicians feel the same way about homocysteine. Related to the current therapy for arteriosclerosis is a theory-of-sorts based loosely on a set of interlocking factors. Most would say that elevated serum cholesterol is the final common pathway. Responding to an earlier article of ours, the director of the Framingham Study, Dr. William Castelli, said, "Cholesterol is still the culprit." Talk to different clinicians and the emphasis on particular risks varies, but the explanatory pattern is the same. The current theory-of-sorts is so evasive it can't be proved and it is so elastic it can't be disproved.

Ultimately, it is lame. The current multifactorial perspective has not led to an effective cure and it seems unlikely to us that it will. In a powerful but obscure way, one's viewpoint on a problem can block discovery of the solution. This is a subtle and important point to consider with regard to the challenge of curing arteriosclerosis.

LACK OF INTEREST IN THE THEORY

The homocysteine theory is sufficiently distant from the mainstream to be excluded by those researchers enmeshed in the current framework. Medicine, like all science, is a social enterprise. We attended a recent meeting of nutritional investigators interested in arteriosclerosis. At an informal gathering, someone asked what were the current hot research areas. There was some nervous laughter when someone else answered, "Whatever N.I.H. [the National Institutes of Health] is funding." The people who do the research and the people who fund the research are the same people. That isn't a dark conspiracy but a social fact. Any community, no matter how benign, can get into a rut that leads to asking and reasking the same questions.

In addition, the homocysteine theory is loosely linked to the earlier age of vitamins, long out of fashion. In developed countries medical doctors rarely, if ever, see cases of clinical vitamin deficiency and have little need to think about vitamins. It seems far-fetched that a vitamin discovered 45 years ago and seemingly well understood could be related to a disease that accounts for 50 percent of our dead. Also, medically, vitamin therapy has become tainted because their use has been advocated by fringe therapists and outright opportunists with interests more economic than medical.

Physicians also regard vitamins with some amount of wariness, as though they worked as a powerful lure for otherwise legitimate investigators. Linus Pauling is a brilliant chemist but his belief in the therapeutic use of high intakes of vitamin C has been harshly criticized. The high public visibility of the proposition and the stridency of critics insures that physicians and scientists, whether or not they have reviewed the evidence, will associate vitamins with controversy. Whether he is ultimately proven correct, his case is based on clinical and scientific studies. Other vitamin advocates who have done less work and made more claims have suggested particular vitamin cures of everything from cancer (Laetrile, not a vitamin, is called vitamin B_{17}!) to impotence. Vitamin therapy faces a climate of suspicion and physicians are understandably skeptical. The *zeitgeist* affects the homocysteine theory.

Even an intrinsically simple theory, such as the homocysteine theory, is assembled by drawing pieces from studies to build a new kind of perception and understanding. Although McCully united the work of homocystinuria, dietary protein, and vitamin B_6 deficiency into a comprehensible whole, his own research findings, if not read in the light of the homocysteine theory, appear to have little connection to other research in arteriosclerosis.

The homocysteine theory is a new paradigm for explaining arteriosclerotic disease. For a time, until the old patchwork can be expanded to take homocysteine into account or until the homocysteine theory becomes the new mainstream, most relevant facts in the field can have two interpretations, suggesting different lines of experimentation. To date, because few people accept the perspective of the homocysteine theory, and even fewer such people work on the councils awarding research funds, no major investigations inspired by the theory and aimed at testing it have been done. Slow initial phases are common for testing new theories. Clinical medicine must rely on tests that require major commitments of personnel, organization, and time. Such tests will likely follow, particularly as more contradictions arise in the cholesterol hypothesis. The persistence of the cholesterol hypothesis seems to lie in the inertia of daily practice, not in any objective deficiencies of the homocysteine theory as an alternative.

WHAT NEXT?

We suggest that the next step is to study old people. We know that most old people have very low blood levels of vitamin B_6 and a high incidence of severe arteriosclerosis. The concentration of homocysteine is measurable; if researchers find that it is high in old people, it would be vital to see if daily supplements of vitamin B_6 can reduce residual homocysteine and also reduce the incidence of coronary attacks.

It is also important to carry out long-term studies like the Framingham study—starting with younger people, then following their progress. Wilcken and Wilcken found that there was a considerable range of serum homocysteine levels in the blood of "normal" people after a methionine load. Are those people with higher homocysteine levels at higher risk of showing clinical effects later? If so, can the risk be reversed? These kinds of questions could be addressed in such long-term studies.

It is necessary to study the cellular means by which homocysteine leads to arteriosclerosis, then determine the protective effects of vitamin B_6. This would clarify and define the limits of therapeutic intervention.

It is not difficult to measure serum homocysteine and serum vitamin B_6 in the clinical laboratory. The only real obstacle would be choice of priorities. If these tests are felt to be important, they can be done.

IF THE THEORY IS CORRECT

In this book, we have concentrated on the arguments related to how homocysteine can cause arteriosclerosis. But we have not yet discussed a major implication—what if the theory is right? Franz J. Inglefinger (1978), editor emeritus of the *New England Journal of Medicine,* points out that the elimination of one cause of death gives opportunity to another cause. "Therapeutic success, in a way, thus fertilizes the ground for failure." Sudden death by coronary attack is perhaps a fate to be preferred over other lingering ailments. But sudden death is not the only possible outcome of arteriosclerosis. Arteriosclerotic impairment of circulation can affect any organ of the body; it is particularly tragic, frustrating, and painful when it affects the brain and causes strokes, resulting in long-term debilitation, loss of independence, and enormous financial burden.

Elimination of arteriosclerotic disease does not mean elimination of death, but it could mean postponement of death. The immediate effect would be a reduction of medical expenditures, just as preventing polio eliminated the expensive care of treating polio victims (iron lungs, therapists, hospital beds, nurses). In the long run, elimination of arteriosclerosis could result in a greater proportion of older people in our society. If in the future, older people who are still productive are not usefully employed by society, then, as Gio Gori and Brian Richter point out, this will have a "recessive economic potential." It does not necessarily have to be this way. But it is difficult to say what changes will occur. Gori and Richter point out that since 1900 there has been only a small increase in the life expectancy of white males over age 30. A society that has a higher proportion of older people will have a different outlook, a different style. Perhaps the recent increase in the age for mandatory retirement is a harbinger of things to come.

SOFTENING OF ARTERIES?

It is perhaps possible that homocysteine-generated arteriosclerosis, once it has become severe enough, cannot be reversed and worsens progressively. We are fairly sanguine, however, because of the work during World War II which showed that it was possible to have huge drops in coronary heart disease in a relatively short period. Although the evidence is not yet convincing that vitamin B_6 will soften arteries, we behave as though it were a reasonable possibility and minimally, it might prevent the worsening of arterial disease. In 1977 Dr. Fumio Kuzuya of Nagoya University published a short paper showing that arteriosclerosis induced by vitamin B_6 deficiency in monkeys can be reversed by adding pyridoxine to the diet. He found that when vitamin B_6 was given therapeutically, the coronary arteries in particular "showed a very rapid recovery, specifically having a strong reversibility."

In addition, Dr. Moses Suzman, a cardiologist in Johannesburg, South Africa, published an abstract in 1973 in which he described work on 17 patients with coronary artery disease. All had abnormal electrocardiograms and 12 suffered angina. He reduced the animal protein (because of its high methionine content) in the patients' diets to between one-fourth and one-half what it had been. Each patient took 100 mg of pyridoxine a day in addition to other B vitamins. After an average of 13 months, the electrocardiograms became less abnormal and some even became normal. Those with angina had complete or partial relief. Dr. Suzman suggested that his results warranted controlled trials. We concur.

When we began writing this book, we were curious but relatively neutral regarding the validity of the theory we intended to examine. Now, after much searching, we are no longer quite so dispassionate. Both of us now believe the theory is strong and internally consistent. Despite our long-standing hesitancy regarding vitamins, we both now take supplements of vitamin B_6. We haven't become vegetarians, but we do eat smaller portions of animal protein.

If you are cautious, you can hedge your bets. Following the advice emerging from the homocysteine theory to choose a diet lower in protein and higher in vitamin B_6 does not preclude simultaneous use of other strategies. Although the cholesterol hypothesis is apparently invalid, no one will be hurt by following a low-cholesterol diet as well.

Finally, if you have followed us this far, you will probably agree that arteriosclerosis is a fascinating puzzle. The picture we have presented, although still not completely formed, makes us optimistic about our ability to understand and control the disease.

We began our book with a quotation from David Hume on how we become habituated to certain connections which appear to demonstrate cause and effect. He later wrote (perhaps after studying arteriosclerosis?):

> Twou'd be very happy for men in the conduct of their lives and actions, were the same objects always conjoin'd together, and we had nothing to fear but the mistakes of our own judgment, without having any reason to apprehend the uncertainty of nature. But as 'tis frequently found, that one observation is contrary to another, and that cause and effects follow not in the same order, of which we have had experience, we are oblig'd to vary our reasoning on account of this uncertainty, and take into consideration the contraiety of events.

Glossary

adventitia outer layer of arterial wall.

amino acid small acidic molecule which contains an amino group of one nitrogen atom and two hydrogen atoms. Usually used as a building block of protein.

aneurysm a weakened area of a blood vessel which tends to balloon out.

angina pain, usually in the chest.

angina pectoris spasmodic pains in the chest usually due to lack of oxygen in heart tissue.

arteriosclerosis hardening and thickening of arteries by a variety of means.

atheroma a plaque of thickened tissue in the intima. It contains smooth muscle cells and deposits of cholesterol and other lipids.

atherosclerosis form of arteriosclerosis leading to atheromas.

calcification deposition of calcium salts onto tissue. Tends to harden the tissue.

carbohydrates molecules such as sugars, starches, and celluloses which contain carbon, hydrogen, and oxygen. The latter two atoms are usually present in the same proportion as in water. Carbohydrates can be classified as simple and complex depending on the structure of the molecules.

cholesterol a fatty substance used as a building block in all animal cells. It is also found in atheromas.

cholesterolemia a high level of cholesterol in the blood.

co-enzyme a small molecule required for the functioning of certain enzymes. Vitamin B_6 is a co-enzyme.

cystathionine amino acid produced by homocysteine metabolism.

endothelium single layer of cells that in normal arteries lines the inside of the arterial wall.

enzyme a protein that speeds up (catalyzes) a specific chemical reaction.

fibromusculoelastic lesion a plaque containing a proliferation of smooth muscle cells and connective tissue but little or no cholesterol or other lipids.

fibrous plaque an atheroma.

homocysteic acid a form of homocysteine.

homocysteine an amino acid formed by the metabolism of methionine. Not usually found in protein, it is very toxic to arterial walls.

homocystine an amino acid readily formed (oxidized) from two homocysteine molecules. In vitamin B_6 deficiency there are high levels of homocystine in the urine.

homocystinemia high level of homocystine in the urine.

homocystinuria high level of homocystine in the blood.

hypertension high blood pressure.

internal elastic lamina a thin sheet of elastic fibers next to the endothelium.

intima inner layer of arterial wall made up of the endothelium and internal elastic lamina.

ischemic lacking in blood due to obstruction or constriction of blood vessel.

lamina a thin layer.

lipids organic substances, including cholesterol, that are insoluble in water but dissolve in fat solvents.

lipoprotein a combination of lipid and protein that is soluble in blood.
   high-density (HDL) contains a greater proportion of protein.
   low-density (LDL) contains a lesser proportion of protein.

lumen the hollow part of the artery.

media middle layer of arterial wall.

metabolism the transformation of molecules into other molecules within the body.

methionine a sulfur-containing amino acid found in food protein.

myocardial infarction damage to heart tissue due to obstruction of blood flow to that tissue.

placebo an inactive substance given to patients and used as a control to study other substances.

plaque a patch of artery containing abnormal tissue.

polyunsaturated fat fat molecules which may add extra atoms to their structure.

protein molecule composed of amino acids.

proteoglycan molecule molecule made of sugar and protein.

pyridoxal another form of vitamin B_6. Also heat sensitive.

pyridoxal phosphate the active (co-enzyme) form of vitamin B_6. Made in the body from pyridoxine, pyridoxal or pyridoxamine.

pyridoxamine a form of vitamin B_6. Heat sensitive.

pyridoxine a form of vitamin B_6. More stable than pyridoxal and pyridoxamine.

saturated fat fat molecules which can not add more atoms to their structure. Tend to be solid at room temperature.

serum cholesterol cholesterol in the blood.

smooth muscle type of muscle cell found in the arterial wall. In atherosclerosis smooth muscle cells move from media to intima.

thrombosis aggregation of blood elements which may obstruct flow of blood.

xanthurenic acid an acid produced and urinated in abnormally large quantities under vitamin B_6 deficiency.

Bibliography

Adams, P. W., Rose, D. P., Folkard, J., Wynn, V., Strong, R., and Seed, M. 1973. Effect of pyridoxine hydrochloride (vitamin B_6) upon depression associated with oral contraception. Lancet 1: 897–904.

Anitschkow, N. 1933. Experimental arteriosclerosis in animals. In *Arteriosclerosis*, ed. E. V. Cowdry, New York: Macmillan.

Anitschkow, N. 1967. A history of experimentation on arterial atherosclerosis in animals. In *Cowdry's Arteriosclerosis*, 2d ed., ed. H. T. Blumenthal, Springfield: Charles C. Thomas.

Arthaud, B. 1970. Cause of death in 339 Alaskan natives as determined by autopsy. Arch. Path. 90: 433–438.

Baker, E. M., Canham, J. E., Nunes, W. T., Sauberlich, H. E., and McDowell, M. E. 1964. Vitamin B_6 requirement for adult men. Amer. J. Clin. Nutr. 15: 59–66.

Bauernfeind, J. C., and Miller, O. N. 1978. Vitamin B_6: nutritional and pharmaceutical usage, stability, bioavailability, antagonists, and safety. In *Human vitamin B_6 requirements*. Washington, D. C.: National Academy of Sciences.

Benditt, E. P., and Benditt, J. M. 1973. Evidence for a monoclonal origin of human atherosclerotic plaques. P. N. A. S. 70: 1753–1756.

Borsook, H. 1964. The relation of the vitamin B_6 requirement to the amount in the diet. Vitamins and Hormones 22: 855–874.

Boxer, G. E., Pruss, M. P., and Goodhart, R. S. 1957. Pyridoxal-5-phosphoric acid in whole blood and isolated leukocytes of man and animals. J. Nutr. 63: 623–636.

Bunting, W. R. 1965. The stability of pyridoxine added to cereals. Cereal Chem. 42: 569–572.

Burton, R. F. 1863. *Abeokuta and the Camaroons Mountains. An Exploration*. London: Tinsley Brothers.

Canham, J. E., Nunes, W. T., and Eberlin, E. W. 1964. Electroencephalographic and central nervous system manifestations of B_6 deficiency and induced B$_6$ dependency in normal human adults. Proc. VI International congress Nutr.: 537.

Carson, N. A. J., and Carre, I. J. 1969. Treatment of homocystinuria with pyridoxine. A preliminary study. Arch. Dis. Childhd. 44: 387–392.

Carson, N. A. J., Cusworth, D. C., Dent, C. E., Field, C. M. B., Neill, D. W., and Westall, R. G. 1963. Homocystinuria: a new inborn error of metabolism associated with mental deficiency. Arch. Dis. Childhd. 38: 425–436.

Carson, N. A. J., Dent, C. E., Field, C. M. B., and Gaull, G. E. 1965. Homocystinuria clinical and pathological review of 10 cases. J. Pediat. 66: 565–583.

Carson, N. A. J., and Neill, D. W. 1962. Metabolic abnormalities detected in a survey of mentally backward individuals in Northern Ireland. Arch. Dis. Childhd. 37: 505–513.

Castelli, W. P. et al. 1977. HDL cholesterol and other lipids in coronary heart disease. The cooperative lipoprotein phenotyping study. Circulation 55: 767–772.

Cerecedo, L. R., and De Renzo, E. C. 1950. Protein intake and vitamin B$_6$ deficiency in the rat III. The effect of supplementing a low-protein vitamin B$_6$ deficient diet with tryptophan and with other sulfur-free amino acids. Arch. Biochem. 29: 273–280.

Chung, A. S. M., Pearson, W. N., Darby, W. J., Miller, O. N., and Goldsmith, G. A. 1961. Folic acid, vitamin B$_6$, pantothenic acid, and vitamin B$_{12}$ in human dietaries. Am. J. Clin. Nutr. 9: 573–582.

Church, C. F., and Church, H. N. 1975. *Food Values of Portions Commonly Used*. Philadelphia: J. B. Lippincott.

Clarkson, S., and Newburgh, L. H. 1926. The relation between atherosclerosis and ingested cholesterol in the rabbits. J. Exp. Med. 43: 595–612.

Cleary, R. E., Lumeng, L., and Li, T. K. 1975. Maternal and fetal plasma levels of pyridoxal phosphate at term: adequacy of vitamin B$_6$ supplementation during pregnancy. Am. J. Obstet. Gynecol. 121: 25–28.

Cohen, P. A., Schneidman, K., Ginsberg-Fellner, F., Sturman, J. A., Knittle, J., and Gaull, G. E. 1973. High pyridoxine diet in the rat: possible implications for megavitamin therapy. J. Nutr. 103: 143–151.

Connor, W. E., Stone, D. B., and Hodges, R. E. 1964. The interrelated effects of dietary cholesterol and fat upon human serum lipid levels. J. Clin. Invest. 43: 1691–1696.

Contractor, S. F., and Shane, B. 1970. Blood and urine levels of vitamin B$_6$ in the mother and fetus before and after loading of the mother with vitamin B$_6$. Am. J. Obstet. Gynecol. 107: 635–640.

Coronary Drug Project. 1975. Clofibrate and niacin in coronary heart disease. JAMA 231: 360–381.

Coursin, D. B. 1955. Symposium on frontiers of human nutrition in relation to milk: vitamin B₆ (pyridoxine) in milk. Quart. Rev. Pediat. 10: 2–9.

CRC 1972. *Handbook of Food Additives*. 2d ed. Cleveland: CRC Press.

Davis, Adele. 1970. *Let's Eat Right to Keep Fit*, New York: New American Library.

del Pozo, E., and Brun del Re, R. 1979. Vitamin B₆ in nursing mothers. N. E. J. Med. 301: 107.

Donahue, S., Sturman, J. A., and Gaull, G. E. 1974. Arteriosclerosis due to homocyst(e)inemia. Failure to reproduce the model in weanling rabbits. Am. J. Path. 77: 167–174.

Driskell, J. A., Geders, J. M, and Urban, M. C. 1976. Vitamin B₆ status of young men, women and women using oral contraceptives. J. Lab. Clin. Med. 87: 813–821.

Duff, G. L. 1935. Experimental cholesterol arteriosclerosis and its relationship to human arteriosclerosis. Arch. Path. 20: 81–123; 259–304.

Ejderhamn, J., and Hamfelt, A. 1980. Pyridoxal phosphate concentration in blood in newborn infants and their mothers compared with the amount of extra pyridoxol taken during pregnancy and breast feeding. Acta Paediatr. Scand. 69: 327–330.

El-Zoghby, S. M., El-Shafei, A. K., Abdel-Tawab, G. A., and Kelada, F. S. 1970. Studies on the effect of reserpine therapy on the functional capacity of the tryptophan-niacin pathway in smoker and non-smoker males. Biochem. Pharmacol. 19: 1661–1667.

Enos, W. F., Holmes, R. H., and Beyer, J. 1953. Coronary disease among United States soldiers killed in action in Korea. JAMA 152: 1090–1093.

Feldman, S. A., Ho, K. J., Lewis, L. A., Mikkelson, B., and Taylor, C. B. 1972. Lipid and cholesterol metabolism in Alaskan Arctic Eskimos. Arch. Path. 94: 42–58.

Finlayson, R. 1965. Spontaneous arterial disease in exotic animals. J. Zool. 147: 239–343.

Flynn, M. A., Nolph, G. B., Flynn, T. C., Kahrs, R., and Krause, G. 1979. Effect of dietary egg on human serum cholesterol and triglycerides. Amer. J. Clin. Nutr. 32: 1051–1057.

Fox, H. 1933. Arteriosclerosis in lower animals and birds. In *Arteriosclerosis*, ed. E. V. Cowdry, New York: Macmillan.

Frank, G. C., Berenson, G. S., and Webber, L. S. 1978. Dietary studies and the relationship of diet to cardiovascular disease risk factor variables in 10 year old children: the Bogalusa heart study. Am. J. Clin. Nutr. 31: 328–340.

Franz, D. N. 1975. Drugs for Parkinson's disease: centrally acting muscle relaxants. In *The Pharmacological Basis of Therapeutics*. 5th ed., eds. L. S. Goodman, and A. Gilman, New York: Macmillan.

Friedman, M., Rosenman, R., and Byers, S. 1955. Deranged cholesterol metabolism and its possible relationship to human atherosclerosis: a review. J. Geront. 10: 60–85.

Fuster, V., Frye, R. L., Connolly, D. C., Danielson, M. A., Elueback, L. R., and Kurland, L. T. 1975. Arteriographic patterns early in the onset of the coronary syndromes. Brit. Heart J. 37: 1250–1255.

Gaull, G. E., Rassin, D. K., and Sturman, J. A. 1969. Enzymatic and metabolic studies of homocystinuria: effects of pyridoxine. Neuropaediatrie 1: 199–226.

Geigy 1970. *Scientific Tables*, 7th ed., Ardsley, N.Y.: Geigy.

Gerritsen, T., Vaughn, J. G., and Waisman, H. A. 1962. The identification of homocystine in the urine. Biochem. Biophys. Res. Commun. 9: 493–496.

Gibson, J. B., Carson, N. A. J., and Neill, D. W. 1964. Pathological findings in homocystinuria. J. Clin. Path. 17: 427–437.

Glueck, C. J., Mattson, F., and Bierman, E. L. 1978. Diet and coronary heart disease: another view. N. E. J. Med. 298: 1471–1474.

Gori, G. B., and Richter, J. 1978. Macroeconomics of disease prevention in the United States. Science 200: 1124–1130.

Gottman, A. W. 1960. A report of 103 autopsies on Alaskan natives. Arch. Path. 70: 117–124.

Greengard, P. 1975. Water-soluble vitamins. In *The Pharmacological Basis of Therapeutics*. eds. L. S. Goodman, and A. Gilman, 5th ed., New York: Macmillan.

Greentree, L. B. 1979. Dangers of vitamin B_6 in nursing mothers. N.E.J. Med. 300: 141–142.

Groen, J. J., Baloch, M., Levy, M., and Yaron, E. 1964. Nutrition of the Bedouin in the Negev Desert. Amer. J. Clin. Nutr. 14: 37–46.

Groom, D. 1967. The use of population statistics in the study of etiologic factors. In *Cowdry's Arteriosclerosis*, ed. H. T. Blumenthal, Springfield: Charles C. Thomas.

Gruberg, E. R., and Raymond, S. A. 1979. Beyond cholesterol, a new theory on arteriosclerosis. The Atlantic 243: no. 5, 59–65.

Gvozdova, L. G., Paramonova, E. G., Goryachenkova, E. V., and Polyakova, L. A. 1966. Sodyerzhania pyridoksalyevich kofermentov v plazmye bolnich koronarnim atyerosklerozom na fonye lechibnoi diyeti i poslye dopolnitelnovo priyema vitamina B_6 [The level of pyridoxalic co-enzymes in the plasma of patients with coronary atherosclerosis kept on a curative diet and after an additional intake of vitamin B$_6$]. Voprosy Pitanyia 25: 40–44.

Gyorgy, P. 1934. Vitamin B$_2$ and the pellagra-like dermatitis in rats. Nature 133: 498–499.

Gyorgy, P. 1971. Developments leading to the metabolic role of vitamin B$_6$. Am. J. Clin. Nutr. 24: 1250–1256.

Hamfelt, A. 1964. Age variation of vitamin B$_6$ metabolism in man. Clin. Chem. Acta 10: 48–54.

Harding. R. S., Plough, I. C., and Friedmann, T. E. 1959. The effect of storage on the vitamin B$_6$ content of a packaged army ration, with a note on the human requirement for the vitamin. J. Nutr. 68: 323–332.

Harker, L. A., Ross, R., Slichter, S. J., and Scott, C. R. 1976. Homocystine-induced arteriosclerosis: the role of endothelial cell injury and platelet response in its genesis. J. Clin. Invest. 58: 731–741.

Harker, L. A., Slichter, S. J., Scott, C. R., and Ross, R. 1974. Homocystinemia: vascular injury and arterial thrombosis. N. E. J. Med. 291: 537–543.

Harris, S. A., Harris, E. E., and Burg, R. W. 1968. Pyridoxine. In, Encyclopedia of Chemical Technology 16: 806–824, New York: Wiley.

Hodkinson, H.M., and Exton Smith, A.N. 1976. Factors predicting mortality in the elderly in the community. Age and Ageing 5: 110–115.

Holtz, P., and Palm, D. 1964. Pharmacological aspects of vitamin B$_6$. Pharmacol. Rev. 16: 113–178.

Horrobin, D. F., et al. 1979. The nutritional regulation of T lymphocyte function. Medical Hypotheses 5: 969–985.

Hume, D. 1967. A treatise of human nature. London: Oxford Univ. Press.

Hunt Jr., A. D. 1957. Abnormally high pyridoxine requirement—summary of evidence suggesting relation between this finding and clinical pyridoxine "deficiency." Am. J. Clin. Nutr. 5: 561–565.

Hunt Jr., A. D., Stokes Jr., J., McCrory, W. W., and Stroud, H. H. 1954. Pyridoxine dependency: report of a case of intractable convulsions in an infant controlled by pyridoxine. Pediatrics 13: 140–144.

Ignatovski, A. I. 1908. Influence de la nourriture animale sur l'organisme des lapins. Arch. Med. Exp. 20: 1–20.

———— 1908. Izminechia parenchymatoznich organach y vo aort crolykov pod vliyaniyem shibotnavo bilka. St. Petersburg Voennomeditsinskai akkademiie. Izvestiya imperatorskoi xvii: 231–244.

———— 1909. Uber die wirkung des tierischen eiweisses auf die aorta und die parenchymatous organe der kaninchen. Virchows Arch. F. Path. Anat. U. Physiol. 198: 248–270.

Inglefinger, F. J. 1978. Medicine: meritorious or meretricious. Science 200. 942–946.

Irey, N. S., Manion, W. C., and Taylor, H. B. 1970. Vascular lesions in women taking oral contraceptives. Arch. Path. 89: 1–8.

Irey, N. S., and Morris, H. J. 1973. Intimal vascular lesions associated with female reproductive steroids. Arch Path. 96: 227–234.

Ismail, A.-E.-A. 1928. Aetiology of hyperpiesis in Egyptians. Lancet 2: 275–277.

Jaffe, D., Hartroft, W. S., Manning, M., and Eleta, G. 1971. Coronary arteries in newborn children: intimal variations in longitudinal sections and their relationships to clinical and experimental data. Acta Paediat. Scand. Suppl. 219.

Jick, H., Dinan, B., Herman, R., and Rothman, K. J. 1978. Myocardial infarction and other vascular diseases in young women. JAMA 246: 2548–2552.

Jolliffe, N., and Archer, M. 1959. Statistical associations between international coronary heart disease rates and certain environmental factors. J. Chron. Dis. 9: 636–652.

Kahn, H. A., Medalie, J. H., Neufeld, N. H., Riss, E., Balogh, M., and Groen, J. J. 1969. Serum cholesterol: its distribution and association with dietary and other variables in a survey of 10,000 men. Isr. J. Med. Sci. 5: 1117–1127.

Kannel, W. B., and Gordon, T. eds. 1970. The Framingham study. An epidemiological investigation of cardiovascular disease. Section 24: The Framingham diet study: diet and the regulation of serum cholesterol. U.S. Government Printing Office.

Kannel, W. B., McGee, D., and Gordon, T. 1976. A general cardiovascular risk profile: the Framingham study. Am. J. Cardiol. 38: 46–51.

Karlin, M. R. 1959. Effet d'un enrichissement en pyridoxine sur la teneur en vitamin B_6 du lait de femme. Bull. Soc. Chem. Biol. 41: 1085–1091.

Kerr, W. K., Barkin, M., Levers, P. E., Woo, S. K.-C., and Menczyk, Z. 1965. The effect of cigarette smoking on bladder carcinogens in man. Can. Med. Assoc. J. 93: 1–7.

Kertesz, Z. I. 1966. Food and food-processing. In *Encyclopedia of Chemical Technology* 10: 23–61, New York: John Wiley.

Keys, A. 1975. Coronary heart disease—the global picture. Atherosclerosis 22: 149–192.

Keys, A., Kimura, N., Kusukawa, A., Bronte-Stewart, B., Larsen, N. P., and Keys, M. H. 1958. Lessons from serum cholesterol studies in Japan, Hawaii and Los Angeles. Ann. Intern. Med. 48: 83–94.

Kirschmann, J. D. 1975. *Nutrition Almanac*. New York: McGraw-Hill.

Kuzuya, F. 1977. Reversibility of atherosclerosis in pyridoxine-deficient monkeys. In *Atherosclerosis IV*. eds. G. Schettler, Y. Goto, Y. Hata, and G. Klose, Berlin: Springer-Verlag.

Kuzuya, H. 1959. Arteriosclerosis in pyridoxine deficient monkeys. J. Primatol. 2: 99.

Leon, A. S., Spiegel, H. E., Thomas, G., and Abrams, W. D. 1971. Pyridoxine antagonism of levodopa in Parkinsonism. JAMA 218: 1924–1927.

Lepkovsky, S., Roboz, E., and Haagen-smit, A. J. 1943. Xanthurenic acid and its role in the tryptophane metabolism of pyridoxine-deficient rats. J. Biol. Chem. 149: 195–201.

Levene, C. I. 1978. Atherosclerosis—disease of old age or infancy? J. Clin. Path. 31: Suppl. (Roy. Coll. Path.) 165–173.

Levy, J. V., and Bach y Rita, P. 1976. *Vitamins: Their Use and Abuse*. New York: Liveright.

Liebling, A. J. 1964. *The Press*. New York: Ballantine Books.

Long, E. R. 1967. Development of our knowledge of arteriosclerosis. In *Cowdry's Arteriosclerosis*, ed. H. T. Blumenthal, Springfield: Charles C. Thomas.

Lowe, C. V., et al. 1966. American Academy of Pediatrics Committee on Nutrition. Vitamin B_6 requirements in man. Pediatrics 38: 1068–1076.

Lushbough, C. H., Weichmen, J. M., and Schweigert, B. S. 1959. The retention of vitamin B_6 in meat during cooking. J. Nutr. 67: 451–459.

Mahler, H. R., and Cordes, E. H. 1971. *Biological chemistry* 2d ed. New York: Harper and Row.

Mann, G. V. 1968. Blood changes in experimental primates fed purified diets: pyridoxine and riboflavin deficiency. Vitamins and Hormones 26: 465–485.

Mann, G. V. 1977. Diet-Heart: End of an era. N. E. J. Med. 297: 644–650.

Mann, G. V., and Andrus, S. B. 1956. Xanthomatosis and atherosclerosis produced by diet in an adult Rhesus monkey. J. Lab. Clin. Med. 48: 533–556.

Mann, G. V., Andrus, S. B., McNally, A., and Stare, F. J. 1953. Experimental atherosclerosis in Cebus monkeys. J. Exp. Med. 98: 195–218.

Mason, J. K. 1963. Asymptomatic disease of coronary arteries in young men. Brit. Med. J. 2: 1234–1237.

McCance, R. A. 1962. Food, growth and time. Lancet 2: 621–626.

McCully, K. S. 1969. Vascular pathology of homocysteinemia: implications for the pathogenesis of arteriosclerosis. Am. J. Path. 56: 111–128.

McCully, K. S. 1970. Importance of homocysteine-induced abnormalities of proteoglycan structure in arteriosclerosis. Am. J. Path. 59: 181–193.

McCully, K. S. 1972. Homocysteinemia and arteriosclerosis. Am. Heart. J. 83: 571–573.

McCully, K. S., and Ragsdale, B. D. 1970. Production of arteriosclerosis by homocysteinemia. Am. J. Path. 61: 1–11.

McMichael, J. 1976. Prevention of coronary heart-disease. Lancet 2: 569.

McNamara, J. J., Molot, M. A., Stremble, J. F., and Cutting, R. T. 1971. Coronary artery disease in combat casualties in Vietnam. JAMA 216: 1185–1187.

Meeker, D. R., and Kesten, H. D. 1941. Effect of high protein diets on experimental atherosclerosis of rabbits. Arch Path. 31: 147–162.

Mellies, M. J., Ishikawa, T. T., Gartside, P., Burton, K., MacGee, J., Allen, K., Steiner, P. M., Brady, D., and Glueck, C. J. 1978. Effects of varying maternal dietary cholesterol and phytosterol in lactating women and their infants. Amer. J. Clin. Nutr. 71: 1347–1354.

Morrison, A. R. and Sarett, H. P. 1959. Studies on B vitamin interrelationships in growing rats. J. Nutr. 68: 473–484.

Mueller, J. H. 1922. A new sulphur-containing amino acid isolated from casein. Proc. Soc. Exptl. Biol. Med. 19: 161–163.

Mushett, C. W., and Emerson, G. 1956. Arteriosclerosis in pyridoxine-deficient monkeys and dogs. Fed. Proc. 15: 526.

National Academy of Sciences 1974 and 1980. Recommended Dietary Allowances, 8th and 9th eds. Washington, D. C.

National Academy of Sciences 1980. Toward healthful diets. Washington, D. C.

Newburgh, L. H., and Clarkson, S. 1923. The production of atherosclerosis in rabbits by feeding diets rich in meat. Arch. Int. Med. 31: 653–676.

Newburgh, L. H., and Marsh, P. L. 1925. Renal injuries by amino acids. Arch. Int. Med. 36: 682–711.

Nichols, A. B., Ravenscroft, C., Lamphiear, D. E., and Ostrander Jr., L. D. 1976. Independence of serum lipid levels and dietary habits, the Tecumseh study. JAMA 236: 1948–1953.

Nizhegorodov, V. M., and Markhotski, Y. L. 1971. Effect of prolonged combined exposure to carbon monoxide, nitrogen oxide and ammonia on the vitamin B_6 requirement of albino rats. Hyg. Sanit. 36: 137–139 nos. 1–3.

Noakes, T. D., Opie, L. H., Rose, A. G., and Kleynhans, P. H. T. 1979. Autopsy-proved coronary atherosclerosis in marathon runners. N. E. J. Med. 301: 86–89.

Orr, M. L. 1969. *Pantothenic acid, vitamin B*$_6$ *and vitamin B*$_{12}$ *in foods*. Home Econ. Res. Rept. 36. Washington, D. C.: USDA.

Park, Y. K., and Linkswiler, H. 1970. Effect of vitamin B$_6$ depletion in adult man on the excretion of cystathionine and other methionine metabolites. J. Nutr. 100: 110–116.

Porter, M. W., Yamanaka, W., Carlson, S., and Flynn, M. A. 1977. Effect of dietary egg on serum cholesterol and triglyceride of human males. Am. J. Clin. Nutr. 30: 490–495.

Rabinowitch, I. M. 1936. Clinical and other observations on Canadian Eskimos in the eastern arctic. Canadian Med. Assn. J. 34: 487–501.

Ranke, E., Tauber, S. A., Horonick, A., Ranke, B., Goodhart, R. S., and Chow, B. F. 1960. Vitamin B$_6$ deficiency in the aged. J. Gerontol. 15: 41–44.

Rinehart, J. F., and Greenberg, L. D. 1949. Arteriosclerotic lesions in pyridoxine-deficient monkeys. Amer. J. Path. 25: 481–491.

Rinehart, J. F., and Greenberg, L. D. 1956. Vitamin B$_6$ deficiency in the Rhesus monkey with particular reference to the occurrence of atherosclerosis, dental caries, and hepatic cirrhosis. Amer. J. Clin. Nutr. 4: 318–325.

Robertson, O. H., Wexler, B. C, and Miller, B. F. 1961. Degenerative changes in the cardiovascular system of the spawning Pacific salmon (*Oncorhyncus tshawytschia*). Circulation Res. 9: 826–834.

Rose, D. P., Strong, R., Folkard, J., and Adams, P. W. 1973. Erythrocyte aminotransferase activities in women using oral contraceptives and the effects of vitamin B$_6$ supplementation. Am. J. Clin. Nutr. 26: 48–52.

Ross, R., and Glomset, J. A. 1976. The pathogenesis of atherosclerosis. N. E. J. Med. 295: 369–377; 420–425.

Royal College of General Practitioners' Oral Contraception Study 1977. Mortality among oral-contraceptive users. Lancet 2: 727–731.

Ruffer, M. A. 1910. On arterial lesions found on Egyptian mummies (1580 BC –525 AD). J. Path. & Bacteriol. Cambridge XV: 453–462.

Russell, P. F., West, L. S., and Manwell, R. D. 1963. *Practical Malariology*. 2d ed. London: Oxford Univ. Press.

Schimke, R. V., McKusic, V. A., Huang, T., and Pollack. A. D. 1965. Homocystinuria studies of 20 families with 38 affected members. JAMA 193: 711–719.

Schroeder. H. A. 1955. Is atherosclerosis a conditioned pyridoxal deficiency? J. Chron. Dis. 2: 28–41.

Schroeder, H. A. 1971. Losses of vitamins and trace minerals resulting from processing and preservation of foods. Am. J. Clin. Nutr. 24: 562–573.

Scrimshaw, N. S., and Guzman, M. A. 1968. Diet and atherosclerosis. Lab. Invest. 18: 623–628.

Sebrell Jr., W. H. 1964. The importance of vitamin B$_6$ in human nutrition. Vitamins and Hormones 22: 875–884.

Shupack, J. L., Grieco, A. J., Epstein, A. M., Sansaricq, C., and Snyderman, S. E. 1977. Azaribine, homocystinemia and thrombosis. Arch. Dermatol. 113: 1301–1302.

Sinclair, H. M. 1953. Diet of Canadian indians and Eskimos. Proc. Nutr. Soc. 12: 69–82.

Sinnett, P. F., and Whyte, H. M. 1974. Epidemiological studies in a total highland population, Tukisenta, New Guinea: cardiovascular diseases and relevant clinical, electrocardiographic, radiological and biochemical findings. J. Chronic Dis. 26: 265–290.

Spaeth, G. L., and Barber, G. W. 1965. Homocystinuria in a mentally retarded child and her normal cousin. Trans. Amer. Acad. Ophthal. Otolaryng. 69: 912–930.

Stulb, S. C., McDonough, J. R., Greenberg, B. G., and Hames, C. G. 1965. The relationship of nutrient intake and exercise to serum cholesterol levels in white males in Evans County, Georgia. Am. J. Clin. Nutr. 16: 238–242.

Subbarao, K., Kuchibhotla, J., and Kakker, V. V. 1979. Pyridoxal 5-phosphate—A new physiological inhibitor of blood coagulation and platelet function. Biochem. Pharmacol. 28: 531–534.

Suzman, M. M. 1973. Effect of pyridoxine and low animal protein diet in coronary artery disease. Circulation 48: supplement IV, IV–254.

Tarnower, H. T., and Baker, S. S. 1980. *The Complete Scarsdale Medical Diet*. New York: Bantam Books.

Thomas, L. 1978. Profile. in Bernstein, J. The New Yorker, 2 Jan. 27–46.

Thomas, W. A. 1927. Health of a carnivorous race. A study of the Eskimo. JAMA 88: 1559–1560.

Toor, M., Katchalsky, A., Agmon, J., and Allaouf, D. 1960. Atherosclerosis and related factors in immigrants in Israel. Circulation 22: 265–279.

USDA 1963. *Composition of Foods*. Handbook No. 8 Washington, D. C.

USDA 1978. *Composition of Foods - Dairy and egg products*. Handbook no. 8–1, Washington, D. C.

Vartiainen, I., and Kanerva, K. 1947. Arteriosclerosis and war-time. Ann. Med. Int. Fenniae 36: 748–758.

Vesselinovitch, D., Wissler, R. W., Hughes, R., and Borensztajn, J. 1976. Reversal of advanced atherosclerosis in Rhesus monkeys. Atherosclerosis 23: 155–176.

Vessey, M. P., McPherson, K., and Johnson, B. 1977. Mortality among women participating in the Oxford/Family Planning Association contraceptive study. Lancet 2: 731–733.

Vilter, R. W., Mueller, J. F., Glazer, H. S., Jarrold, T., Abraham, J., Thompson, C., and Hawking, V. R. 1953. The effect of vitamin B_6 deficiency induced by desoxypyridoxine in human beings. J. Lab. Clin. Med. 42: 335–357.

Vlodaver, Z., Kahn, H. A., and Neufeld, H. N. 1969. The coronary arteries in early life in three different ethnic groups. Circulation 39: 541–550.

Wade, N. 1980. Food Board's fat report hits fire. Science 209: 248–250.

Whyte, M., Nestel, P., and MacGregor, A. 1977. Cholesterol metabolism in New Guineans. Europ. J. Clin. Invest. 7: 53–60.

Wilcken, D. E. L., and Gupta, V. J. 1979. Cysteine-homocysteine mixed disulphide: differing plasma concentrations in normal men and women. Clin. Sci. 57: 211–216.

Wilcken, D. E. L., and Wilcken, B. 1976. The pathogenesis of coronary artery disease. A possible role for methionine metabolism. J. Clin. Invest. 57: 1079–1082.

Wilson, R. G., and Davis, R. E. 1977. Serum pyridoxal concentrations in children with diabetes mellitus. Pathology 9: 95–98.

Yerushalmy, J., and Hilleboe, H. E. 1957. Fat in the diet and mortality from heart disease. N.Y. J. Med. 57: 2343–2354.

Index